The Essential Amish Handbook to Lifestyle Discipline and Survival Ways Beyond Modern Living:

An Amish Traditional Recipes Cookbook for Wholesome

Challenging Lifestyles

The Essential Amish Handbook to Lifestyle Discipline and Survival Ways Beyond Modern Living

Library of Congress Cataloging-in-Publication Data

Available upon request.

Disclaimer

The information in this book is intended for educational and informational purposes only. It is not a substitute for professional medical advice, diagnosis, or treatment. Always seek the advice of your physician or other qualified health provider with any questions you may have regarding a medical condition or health goals.

Contact Email: mspublishing2003@gmail.com

Cover Design by SHS Publishers

Printed in USA

Contents

Introduction to Ancient Survival Wisdom

The origins of survival techniques trace back thousands of years, where human ingenuity and adaptability played crucial roles in overcoming the formidable challenges of a harsh and unpredictable environment. Long before the convenience of modern technology and established societies, our ancestors relied on a deep connection to the natural world. This primal relationship, cultivated over centuries, allowed them to devise survival strategies that were practical, resourceful, and sustainable. These techniques were born out of necessity as early humans navigated the demands of a world where food sources were seasonal, shelter was fragile, and weather patterns were often hostile. Survival was a daily endeavor, and each technique developed through trial and error, passing on through oral traditions, demonstrating an accumulated body of knowledge that kept communities alive across generations.

Early survival methods were shaped by the geography, climate, and resources available to each group, leading to diverse techniques that adapted to different environments. In dense forests, people became adept at distinguishing edible from poisonous plants, while those in coastal regions learned to navigate waters and harvest fish. The steppe nomads mastered the art of creating mobile homes and shelters, while desert tribes developed unique water conservation strategies. Observing animal behaviors, our ancestors derived early knowledge of weather patterns, seasonal migrations, and natural hazards, all essential to survival in their surroundings. Through these observations, humans learned to track prey, prepare food to avoid spoilage, and craft shelters from natural materials, each skill a survival strategy embedded in the customs and daily lives of ancient communities.

Fire-making was among the most groundbreaking of ancient survival techniques, as it not only provided warmth and protection but also allowed for the cooking and preservation of food. The discovery and mastery of fire is considered a pivotal milestone in human evolution, offering a source of comfort and a means to ward off predators in the dark. Initially, fire was likely obtained from natural sources like lightning strikes. However, with time, our ancestors devised ways to create and maintain fire by striking stones or using friction-based tools such as the hand drill and bow drill. The ability to generate fire transformed the daily life of early humans, enabling them to settle in colder climates and better withstand the elements. Fire was also essential for creating tools from bones and stones, a cornerstone in the technological advancement of early societies that influenced countless other survival techniques.

The development of shelter construction was another fundamental aspect of ancient survival. Shelter offered not only protection from weather and predators but also privacy and comfort. Early humans built shelters using natural resources, often selecting materials that were abundant and easy to manipulate within their specific region. Caves served as some of the earliest forms of shelter, but as populations grew and became more mobile, humans learned to construct structures with wood, mud, grasses, and animal hides. In colder climates, they developed techniques for insulation by creating shelters with thick walls or layering materials to trap heat. Each group developed construction methods suitable for their environment: nomadic tribes built portable tents like yurts and tipis, while settled societies constructed more permanent huts and dwellings. The ability to create shelter directly impacted human survival, as it allowed people to thrive in diverse habitats, from dense jungles to icy tundras.

Foraging for food, another essential survival technique, required vast knowledge of local flora and fauna. Early humans depended heavily on the plant and animal life around them, and over generations, they developed a sophisticated understanding of edible plants, medicinal herbs, and dangerous species to avoid. This knowledge was often encoded in cultural myths, songs, and rituals, preserving it within the community and ensuring it was passed down to future generations. Foraging skills included knowing where to find seasonal fruits and nuts, recognizing signs of animal tracks, and understanding migratory patterns of both animals and birds. This awareness was crucial not only for sustenance but also for medicine, as many plants were used to treat ailments and injuries. The reliance on foraging cultivated a deep respect for nature, as people understood the need to maintain a balance with their environment to ensure future abundance.

Another early survival skill, hunting, required a blend of physical prowess, strategy, and tool-making expertise. Hunting was not only a source of nutrition but also of clothing and materials essential for tool-making. Early humans observed the habits and behaviors of animals, developing sophisticated hunting techniques that often required collective effort and coordination. By crafting rudimentary weapons from stones, bones, and wood, they could take down larger prey, which provided sustenance for extended periods. Tools such as spears, clubs, and later, bows and arrows were designed with an understanding of anatomy, aerodynamics, and material strength. Successful hunts were often ritualized, as they represented the survival of the group, and many societies developed ceremonial practices to honor the animals that sustained them.

The advent of tool-making marked another leap in survival techniques. Initially, tools were simple and improvised, like stones used for cutting or branches fashioned into spears. As humans grew more adept at working with materials, they developed specialized tools for hunting, building, and cooking. Stone tools from the Paleolithic era, such as hand axes and scrapers, are some of the earliest evidence of this ingenuity. The evolution of tool-making over centuries included the transition from stone to bronze and iron, enhancing efficiency and effectiveness. The ability to create and use tools set early humans apart from other species, equipping them with the means to manipulate their environment and secure resources with greater ease. Tool-making extended to the development of containers for storing water and food, which became critical in maintaining supplies for longer periods.

Ancient humans also innovated in areas that may seem surprising, such as early forms of navigation. Navigating using landmarks, the sun, stars, and seasonal changes allowed people to travel great distances, often for trade, migration, or hunting. For early nomadic societies, the skill of navigation was invaluable, as it enabled them to return to familiar territories seasonally or to locate new resources in uncharted areas. Indigenous communities passed down navigational knowledge through stories and oral teachings, creating a living map of their environment that helped them find their way across deserts, mountains, and forests without the need for modern tools like compasses or maps. This spatial awareness contributed to survival by ensuring access to distant food sources and safe passage through unknown terrains.

Water sourcing and purification, too, were pivotal for survival. Ancient humans learned to identify sources of fresh water in rivers, lakes, and even plant roots. Techniques such as sand filtration or boiling were later developments that ensured cleaner drinking water, though in many cases, simply knowing where to find uncontaminated water sources was enough to sustain life. This knowledge became crucial in arid regions where water was scarce, and survival depended on storing and rationing water resources effectively. The necessity of water for survival led to the construction of early water storage systems, which allowed people to maintain a supply even during droughts or periods of scarcity.

These early survival techniques form a tapestry of wisdom and innovation, where each skill was a response to the immediate needs of early humans in an untamed world. The origins of survival techniques reveal a story of adaptation and resilience, showing how, through close observation of nature and a communal approach to knowledge, early humans developed methods that sustained them across millennia. This body of knowledge, though ancient, still serves as a foundation for modern survival strategies and teaches us the importance of living in harmony with the natural world. Understanding these origins allows us to appreciate the endurance of human spirit and adaptability, qualities that remain essential in any era of survival.

Ancient knowledge offers a timeless foundation for modern survival, guiding us in reconnecting with basic skills and the environment in ways that can enhance self-sufficiency, resourcefulness, and resilience. As modern society has grown increasingly dependent on complex systems, from advanced technologies to global supply chains, we've found ourselves removed from basic survival skills that were once integral to human life. However, as natural disasters, power outages, and emergencies continue to occur, there's a rising awareness of the importance of these ancient practices. By revisiting the techniques our ancestors developed, we can enrich our understanding of the natural world, reduce our environmental impact, and gain practical skills that empower us in both ordinary and extraordinary situations.

One of the most significant ways ancient knowledge informs modern survival is through the principle of sustainability. Ancient survival techniques were inherently sustainable, relying on what the environment naturally provided and doing so in a way that minimized waste. Practices such as foraging, hunting, and food preservation were not just survival methods; they were a way of life that allowed early societies to live in harmony with their surroundings. Modern survivalists and preppers often turn to these methods, recognizing the limitations of current agricultural systems and the need for alternative food sources that are less reliant on fossil fuels and other finite resources. Learning to forage for edible plants, preserve food through methods like drying or fermenting, and hunt responsibly provides a level of food security that aligns with ecological balance. These techniques enable people today to build sustainable food sources and reduce dependency on commercial systems, which can be especially critical in times of crisis.

Ancient knowledge also informs modern shelter construction and the use of natural resources. Early humans adapted their shelter designs to fit the climate and geography, creating structures from locally available materials such as wood, mud, stones, or animal skins. In cold regions, they developed insulated shelters, while in warmer climates, they used materials that allowed for ventilation. These ancient shelter-building techniques influence modern practices, particularly in the fields of sustainable architecture and off-grid living. For instance, techniques such as earthen building, cob construction, and passive solar heating are all grounded in ancient methods. By using these age-old principles, people today can create shelters that are energy-efficient, environmentally friendly, and resilient. Moreover, these methods often require less energy and fewer resources than conventional building techniques, making them valuable in a world increasingly conscious of environmental impact.

Fire-making is another fundamental survival skill that highlights the importance of ancient knowledge in the modern context. Fire, which once provided warmth, protection, and a means for cooking, remains a critical survival tool, particularly in wilderness or emergency settings. While modern devices such as lighters and matches make starting a fire easier, understanding friction-based techniques like the bow drill or hand drill can be invaluable if these tools are unavailable. Moreover, the skill of fire management — choosing the right wood, constructing a fire pit, and safely extinguishing flames — harks back to practices that early humans mastered.

In learning these skills, modern survivalists gain an essential tool for situations where electricity or gas is unavailable, such as during extended power outages, wilderness expeditions, or disaster scenarios.

Water sourcing and purification, another critical area, has ancient origins that provide insight into essential techniques still used today. Ancient people learned to locate natural water sources by reading the landscape, watching for signs of water-loving plants, or noting animal trails. They also developed rudimentary purification techniques, such as boiling water or filtering it through sand and gravel. In modern survival situations, these principles are applied to methods like building makeshift filters, understanding which plants can store drinkable water, and reading environmental cues to find water in remote areas. The necessity of these skills becomes apparent when considering the potential for contaminated water sources in emergencies, underscoring the timeless relevance of knowing how to find and purify water using natural resources.

Ancient knowledge of navigation is invaluable in modern survival contexts, especially for those who find themselves without digital tools or maps. Ancient navigators learned to read the stars, the sun's position, and natural landmarks as reliable guides. Indigenous people, in particular, used techniques such as watching the migration patterns of birds or the growth of moss on trees to orient themselves. Today, these skills are essential for wilderness survivalists, military personnel, and anyone interested in outdoor exploration without relying on electronic devices. They offer a sense of direction in remote locations where GPS might fail, and they underscore the importance of spatial awareness and observational skills. In modern survival training, learning ancient navigation techniques fosters a self-reliance that remains relevant even in an age of digital tools.

Furthermore, ancient methods of food preservation continue to provide effective strategies for modern survivalists aiming to create long-lasting, nutritious food supplies. Techniques like fermentation, drying, smoking, and salting were developed long before refrigeration, allowing food to be stored for extended periods. Fermentation, for instance, which was once a common method for preserving vegetables, also introduces beneficial bacteria that support digestive health. Smoking and drying meat allow it to be safely stored without refrigeration, a practice still used in some rural areas and by outdoor adventurers. In today's world, with concerns over food security and potential supply chain disruptions, these preservation techniques offer a low-tech solution for maintaining food supplies that don't depend on electricity or complex equipment.

Ancient medicinal knowledge has also informed modern survival approaches, particularly through the use of natural remedies and herbal medicine. For millennia, people relied on plants to treat ailments, prevent infections, and support general well-being. This knowledge, passed down through generations, allowed early humans to identify beneficial plants and understand their effects. Many modern medicines are derived from plants, such as aspirin from willow bark and quinine from the cinchona tree. Learning about ancient medicinal herbs like garlic, honey, and aloe vera can be vital in situations where modern medical care is inaccessible. Knowing how to create poultices, teas, and salves from natural ingredients provides practical solutions for treating injuries and illnesses, especially in outdoor or remote settings. This herbal knowledge has grown in popularity in modern times as more people seek alternatives to pharmaceuticals, emphasizing the relevance of plant-based healing.

Tool-making, one of the earliest survival techniques, remains essential to modern survival. Ancient people crafted tools from materials available in their environment, such as stones, bones, and wood, creating essential implements for hunting, shelter building, and daily tasks. Even today, understanding the basics of tool-making can be valuable in situations where modern tools are unavailable. Knowing how to fashion a cutting tool from stone or create a makeshift spear from a sturdy branch can enable a person to perform essential survival tasks. In bushcraft and wilderness survival training, these skills are practiced to prepare individuals for situations where they may need to rely solely on their surroundings.

The philosophical aspects of ancient survival also inform modern mindsets. Ancient cultures often fostered a deep respect for nature, viewing survival as a holistic practice that required both physical skills and an understanding of the environment's cycles. This perspective encouraged an attitude of gratitude and conservation, with the knowledge that resources were finite and needed to be carefully managed. Modern survivalists often adopt a similar mindset, recognizing that preparation, adaptability, and respect for nature are essential to thriving in any setting. By adopting this outlook, people today can learn to approach survival with a balanced mindset that appreciates both the challenges and rewards of living in harmony with the natural world.

In essence, ancient knowledge provides modern survivalists with a valuable toolkit for self-sufficiency and adaptability, offering not only practical skills but also insights into sustainability and resilience. Whether through foraging, fire-making, navigation, or herbal medicine, these age-old techniques offer solutions that stand the test of time, proving that our ancestors' methods remain as relevant today as they were thousands of years ago.

Essential Skills for Self-Sufficiency

Shelter Construction with Natural Materials

The construction of shelters using natural materials is an essential skill for self-sufficiency, offering protection from the elements and enabling survival in various environments. For centuries, humans have relied on their surrounding resources to create structures that are both functional and sustainable. The methods and materials vary depending on the environment — from forested regions to open plains, mountains, and deserts. This adaptability is one of the most remarkable aspects of human survival, as each setting offers unique resources and requires specific techniques. Understanding how to build a shelter from natural materials involves not only knowledge of local resources but also a sense of respect for the environment, as ancient and indigenous practices often emphasized using materials in a way that minimized impact on the land.

The primary purpose of a shelter is to provide safety from weather conditions like rain, snow, wind, and extreme temperatures. In colder climates, shelter must offer insulation and a means to trap heat, while in warmer areas, ventilation and shade are more critical. To achieve this balance, ancient and traditional shelters used materials that were abundant, resilient, and suited to their climate. In forested regions, for example, wood and bark are typically accessible and form the primary materials for shelter construction. In contrast, desert dwellers used clay, mud, and stone, while people in grasslands often relied on thatch and tall grasses.

One of the most common traditional shelters is the lean-to, which involves constructing a frame of sturdy branches that leans against a central support, often a tree. This frame is then layered with other materials such as leaves, moss, or bark to create insulation and protection from rain or wind. The lean-to is a versatile structure, as it can be built relatively quickly and requires minimal tools, making it an ideal option in emergency situations. While simple in design, the lean-to demonstrates a key principle of natural shelter construction: utilizing what the environment provides without requiring extensive modification or removal of resources. A lean-to can be built with a single, sloping side to catch heat from a fire, or double-sided for increased protection from harsh winds.

In colder regions, where survival depends on effective insulation, people often construct shelters that can retain warmth, such as igloos or dugouts. Igloos, built by indigenous Arctic communities, are made of compacted snow blocks arranged in a dome shape. Snow, surprisingly, serves as an excellent insulator because of its high air content, which traps heat inside the structure. Inside, temperatures can be significantly warmer than outside, allowing for basic comfort in extreme cold. This technique showcases an understanding of natural materials, as the snow used is packed to a density that offers insulation without melting. Similarly, in forested areas with frigid winters, people may dig into hillsides or create semi-subterranean shelters that use the earth's natural insulation properties to regulate temperature.

In regions where clay and mud are abundant, these materials become the building blocks of shelters that are durable and suitable for a variety of climates. The use of mud bricks, known as adobe, dates back thousands of years and remains a cornerstone of sustainable building practices in arid and semi-arid climates. Adobe bricks are made by mixing clay-rich soil with water and a fibrous material such as straw, which strengthens the mixture as it dries. This blend is poured into molds, shaped into bricks, and left to harden in the sun. Adobe structures are especially effective in warm, dry regions, as their thermal mass keeps interiors cool during the day and warmer at night, regulating indoor temperatures naturally. By working with the earth itself, people can create long-lasting shelters that withstand both heat and drought, making adobe a preferred building method in many traditional communities worldwide.

Thatch and grass-based shelters are another example of ancient construction methods that continue to offer practical solutions, particularly in tropical and subtropical climates. Thatch is made by bundling dried grass, palm fronds, or reeds and layering them to create a waterproof roof or wall. When properly layered, thatch is surprisingly resilient, providing a shelter that is not only waterproof but also breathable, which is essential in hot and humid climates. Indigenous people across Southeast Asia, Africa, and the Americas have long relied on thatch because of its availability and effectiveness. A well-made thatch roof can last for decades and is relatively easy to repair. The use of grass and other plant materials highlights an important principle in natural shelter construction: selecting materials that are renewable and easy to replace, ensuring the shelter remains functional with minimal environmental impact.

Stone is another enduring material for shelter construction, valued for its strength and durability. While gathering and transporting large stones can be labor-intensive, the resulting shelter is sturdy and can last for generations. Stone shelters are common in mountainous regions, where trees may be scarce, but rocks are plentiful. In these areas, people construct shelters by stacking stones in interlocking patterns without mortar, relying on the weight and balance of the stones to hold the structure together. This technique, known as dry stone walling, allows for ventilation through small gaps while providing a solid barrier against wind and rain. In ancient times, the use of stone extended to cave dwellings, where people would find natural formations and adapt them for protection from the elements. Today, stone remains a highly regarded material for sustainable and disaster-resistant building.

An essential part of building with natural materials involves not only selecting the right resources but also adapting the structure to the local environment. Wind direction, sunlight, and the natural contours of the land all influence where and how a shelter should be built. For example, traditional desert shelters are often low to the ground to minimize sun exposure and catch cooling breezes, while forest shelters are elevated to avoid dampness and pests. Ancient builders understood the importance of positioning structures to optimize natural conditions, a principle that modern sustainable architecture continues to embrace. For instance, orienting a shelter to maximize sun exposure during the colder months and minimizing it during the warmer ones can significantly impact its internal temperature, reducing the need for artificial heating or cooling.

The skill of shelter construction with natural materials extends beyond just building techniques; it also encompasses maintenance and repair. Ancient shelters were designed with materials that allowed for regular upkeep. Thatch roofs, for instance, could be patched with new bundles of grass as older sections wore out, and mud walls could be recoated as they eroded from wind and rain. This low-tech maintenance approach ensured that shelters remained functional with minimal expense and effort. Modern natural building practices often borrow from these principles, emphasizing the use of materials that can be sourced locally and easily replaced, reducing the overall ecological footprint of the structure.

Finally, constructing shelters from natural materials teaches important survival values: patience, resilience, and adaptability. Working with raw, unprocessed materials requires an understanding of their properties, such as how wood expands in moisture or how clay hardens in the sun. Each region and climate comes with its own challenges, and learning to build with the available resources fosters a connection with the land. Building a shelter from scratch requires physical effort, resourcefulness, and a level of craftsmanship, which can instill a deep sense of accomplishment and respect for the environment.

In a world that is increasingly embracing sustainable and resilient building methods, shelter construction with natural materials remains not only relevant but also inspiring. It reminds us that self-sufficiency is achievable through knowledge of the natural world and encourages us to look to the wisdom of ancient practices that prioritized environmental balance. Whether for off-grid living, survival training, or reducing our carbon footprint, constructing shelters with natural materials offers a valuable skill set, underscoring the resilience and ingenuity that has allowed humans to thrive in diverse environments for millennia.

The skill of crafting basic tools from natural resources is foundational to self-sufficiency, allowing humans to build shelters, prepare food, hunt, and perform essential survival tasks in the wilderness. Throughout history, people have relied on the resources available in their immediate surroundings to create tools suited to their needs, developing techniques that have been passed down over generations. Learning the art of tool-making from natural materials not only connects us to ancient wisdom but also empowers us to meet basic survival needs without dependence on modern tools. This skill requires creativity, patience, and a keen understanding of the properties of natural resources, each chosen for specific qualities such as durability, sharpness, or flexibility.

Stones are among the oldest materials used in tool-making, and they continue to play a crucial role in survival situations. The first step in crafting stone tools involves selecting the right type of stone; flint, chert, and obsidian are often preferred because of their hardness and ability to be shaped into sharp edges. By carefully striking these stones with harder materials, such as another rock or a piece of antler, one can chip away at the edges to create a sharp, usable point. This technique, known as flintknapping, requires precision and control. The result is a sharp-edged tool suitable for tasks like cutting, scraping, and even hunting. Stone tools made through flintknapping can range from simple hand tools, such as scrapers or cutters, to more complex spear or arrow points used in hunting.

Wood, another abundant and versatile resource, serves as the backbone for various tools due to its strength and flexibility. Branches from hardwood trees, such as oak, hickory, or ash, are ideal for making handles, clubs, digging sticks, and bows. When crafting a handle, it's important to select a piece of wood that is straight and has minimal knots, as this ensures greater strength and durability. The process typically involves peeling off the bark, shaping the wood to fit comfortably in hand, and smoothing out rough edges. For example, a basic digging stick, which can be used to uproot plants, dig fire pits, or forage for edible roots, is created by sharpening one end of a sturdy branch. More sophisticated wooden tools, like bows, require greater skill; the wood must be seasoned, bent, and sometimes reinforced with natural fibers to withstand tension.

Bone and antler are also valuable resources for tool-making, especially in regions where these materials are readily available. Bone tools are strong and can be fashioned into a variety of shapes, including needles, fish hooks, and awls. These items are useful for tasks such as sewing hides, constructing shelters, and crafting traps or nets. To make a bone needle, for example, one would select a long, thin bone, such as a rib, and carefully shape it using stones to scrape and grind it to a fine point. A small hole can be drilled or scraped near the blunt end to create an eye for threading. Bone awls, on the other hand, are pointed tools used for piercing materials such as leather or wood, and they demonstrate how resourceful tool-making allows survivalists to complete tasks that require delicate manipulation, such as making clothing or crafting other tools.

Cordage, or rope, is another critical tool that can be made from natural fibers like plant stems, vines, bark, and animal sinew. Cordage has countless uses in survival settings, including lashing structures together, creating traps or nets, and binding tools securely. To make cordage, one typically harvests materials like inner tree bark (such as from cedar, dogbane, or willow), twists or braids them into strands, and weaves them together for added strength. The twisting process involves separating the fibers and then twisting them tightly while holding them under tension, a method that results in a strong, flexible rope. Sinew, a fiber derived from animal tendons, is incredibly resilient and can be used to make bowstrings, lash arrowheads, and reinforce other tools. By combining fibers from different sources, survivalists can craft ropes of varying thickness and durability, tailored to the demands of specific tasks.

For cutting and scraping tasks, stone and bone tools can be combined with wooden handles to create more sophisticated tools like hatchets and knives. A stone or bone blade is secured to a wooden handle using cordage, sinew, or plant fibers. This process requires careful binding to ensure the blade remains stable during use. For example, to make a stone knife, one would start by crafting a sharp stone blade, then select a sturdy piece of wood for the handle. A notch is carved into the wood to fit the blade snugly, and then the blade is bound to the handle using tightly twisted cordage. The finished tool can be used for preparing food, cutting branches, and even self-defense. This type of composite tool-making showcases how different natural resources can be combined to create versatile, functional implements.

Spears and other hunting tools, essential for obtaining food in the wild, are often made using a combination of wood, stone, and cordage. A simple spear is constructed by attaching a sharpened stone or bone point to a long wooden shaft. The shaft, typically made from a straight branch of hardwood, is stripped of bark, shaped, and often fire-hardened to improve durability. The stone or bone point is securely tied to the end using sinew or natural fiber cordage. In many cases, adhesives made from natural resins or animal fats are used to further secure the binding. Primitive hunters even developed throwing sticks, known as atlatls, which are wooden devices that increase the throwing power of spears. The spear, enhanced by an atlatl, becomes a more effective hunting tool, demonstrating how ancient ingenuity in tool-making can lead to more effective hunting strategies.

Another example of natural tool-making is the construction of traps and snares for capturing small game. These tools, which rely on simple mechanical principles, are often made from materials found in the surrounding environment. For instance, a basic snare trap can be constructed using a loop of cordage tied to a sapling. The sapling is bent over and tied to the snare, so when an animal triggers the trap, the sapling springs up, ensnaring the prey. Another type, the deadfall trap, consists of a heavy object, such as a log or rock, balanced over bait and held in place by a trigger made of sticks. When the animal disturbs the trigger, the object falls, trapping or killing the animal. Both snares and deadfalls showcase how natural resources, combined with a knowledge of animal behavior, can be used to meet basic food needs.

Fire-making tools, perhaps the most critical for warmth, cooking, and protection, are also crafted from natural resources. Techniques like the bow drill and hand drill are ancient methods that use friction to create fire. A bow drill set consists of a spindle (typically made from a straight, dry branch), a fireboard (a flat piece of wood with small notches), a bow, and a socket. The bow is used to rotate the spindle rapidly against the fireboard, generating enough friction to produce a hot ember. Once the ember is created, it is transferred to a tinder bundle — a collection of dry, fibrous material — and gently blown upon to ignite a flame. This tool-making technique requires practice and patience, but it underscores how ancient people used their environment creatively to harness fire without modern ignition tools.

Tool-making from natural resources is not only about survival; it also fosters a deep connection to the environment and an understanding of how to use resources sustainably. By learning to craft tools from what nature provides, survivalists cultivate an appreciation for the skill and ingenuity of ancient people, who thrived without the conveniences of modern technology. Moreover, this practice encourages resourcefulness, adaptability, and patience, as each material requires a different approach and technique. These values are just as important as the tools themselves, reminding us that true self-sufficiency goes beyond mere survival to include a respectful and symbiotic relationship with the natural world.

Mastering basic tool-making from natural resources, therefore, is about more than creating functional objects; it is a journey into understanding our ancestral skills and the deep ingenuity they applied to thrive in the wilderness. In modern times, this skill remains not only valuable for survivalists and outdoor enthusiasts but also inspiring for anyone seeking a closer connection with nature and the empowering knowledge that survival is achievable through simplicity and a profound respect for the environment.

Fire Starting Techniques without Modern Tools

Starting a fire without modern tools is one of the most crucial skills in wilderness survival, providing warmth, protection, a way to cook food, and even a psychological boost. Ancient cultures developed various methods to create fire from natural resources, each suited to different environments and climates. These techniques require understanding the properties of wood, stone, friction, and airflow, and they reflect a deep connection to the land. Although they demand patience and practice, the ability to start a fire without lighters, matches, or other modern conveniences is an empowering skill that connects us to thousands of years of human survival wisdom.

One of the oldest and most widely practiced fire-starting methods is the friction-based technique, which involves creating heat by rubbing two materials together. Among these, the bow drill is one of the most efficient and reliable methods, making it possible to start a fire even in challenging conditions. The bow drill set consists of a spindle, a bow, a fireboard, and a socket. The spindle is a straight, dry stick that will create friction against the fireboard, a flat piece of wood with a small notch where the ember will form. The bow, usually made from a curved branch, holds a cord that wraps around the spindle, allowing for controlled, rapid spinning. As the bow is moved back and forth, the spindle rotates against the fireboard, generating enough heat to produce an ember. Once the ember forms, it's carefully transferred to a tinder bundle, a collection of dry, fibrous materials that can catch and hold the flame.

While the bow drill is effective, it does require some practice and specific materials to be successful. Softwoods, such as cedar, willow, or cottonwood, work best for both the spindle and the fireboard, as they generate heat more easily than hardwoods. The cord for the bow can be crafted from natural materials like rawhide, plant fibers, or even strips of fabric if available. Using the right wood, maintaining steady pressure, and achieving the correct rhythm with the bow are essential for producing the heat required to ignite an ember.

Another popular friction-based method is the hand drill, which, though simpler in construction than the bow drill, requires greater physical endurance. The hand drill uses only a spindle and a fireboard, with the fire-maker placing the spindle between their hands and spinning it rapidly while pressing it against the fireboard. This action generates friction, and with enough speed and pressure, an ember can be created. However, the hand drill requires more skill and strength to maintain the pace and pressure needed to sustain heat, especially over an extended period. It is particularly challenging in cold or damp environments, where maintaining body warmth and energy is crucial. The hand drill works best with softer, dry woods, like those used in the bow drill, and is ideal in regions where suitable wood is plentiful.

The fire plow, another ancient friction method, is often used in tropical and subtropical regions where dense vegetation offers a variety of fire-starting materials. This method involves a fireboard with a groove or channel carved along its length. A pointed stick is rubbed rapidly along this groove, creating friction and producing small particles that ignite into a spark with enough heat. While the fire plow requires less equipment than the bow drill, it demands intense speed and pressure, which can be physically exhausting. It is best used with softer, dry woods and in situations where time and effort can be devoted to creating the fire. Like the hand drill, the fire plow showcases the importance of technique and rhythm in friction-based fire-making, as even slight variations in speed or angle can hinder the process.

In addition to friction methods, the use of flint and steel is another ancient and widely practiced fire-starting technique, dating back to prehistoric times. Flint, chert, or another hard stone is struck against a high-carbon steel object, such as an iron-bearing rock or a specially made piece of steel, producing a spark. This spark is then directed toward a piece of char cloth or tinder fungus, which can hold the heat long enough to ignite a tinder bundle. Flint and steel require less physical energy than friction methods and are especially valuable in wet conditions, as the spark can penetrate damp materials to reach the dry inner layers. This technique relies on understanding the types of stones and metals that produce the best sparks, as well as skill in directing the spark precisely to the tinder.

The concept of solar ignition, another fire-starting method, leverages the power of the sun to create enough heat to ignite a fire. By using a lens, such as a piece of clear glass, ice, or even a polished can lid, one can focus sunlight onto a small point, generating intense heat. When focused on a tinder bundle, this concentrated heat can create an ember that will ignite into a flame. The solar ignition method is highly effective on sunny days and requires little physical exertion, making it an excellent choice when other methods are challenging or unavailable. However, it is weather-dependent and requires both the knowledge of how to focus light effectively and an understanding of where to find or make a lens from available materials.

Another fascinating fire-starting method is the use of chemical reactions found in natural materials. Pyrite, or fool's gold, was used by some ancient cultures in combination with flint to create sparks. When struck together, the pyrite and flint produce a spark that, like in the traditional flint and steel method, can ignite tinder. This technique illustrates an understanding of the properties of minerals and their interactions. In some cases, certain fungi, like horse hoof fungus, can be dried and used as tinder because they smolder easily and can hold an ember for extended periods. These biological resources demonstrate that fire-making is not only about creating sparks but also about finding materials that sustain heat long enough to build a fire.

Tinder selection is equally vital in fire-starting, as it directly influences how quickly and easily the fire catches. Tinder refers to any material that can ignite quickly and burn hot enough to sustain a flame. Natural options include dry grasses, shredded bark, cotton-like seed heads from plants, and fibrous materials like cattail down. In wetter climates, dry inner bark from trees like cedar or birch is often stripped and shredded into fine fibers to create tinder. Char cloth, a fabric that has been partially burned in the absence of oxygen, is another excellent tinder material and can be made by heating cotton cloth inside a metal container until it carbonizes. Once an ember is transferred to the tinder, gently blowing on it can help the fire spread, emphasizing the delicate balance of patience and control needed in fire-making.

Understanding the environmental conditions is another aspect of traditional fire-starting wisdom. Dry, windy conditions provide natural airflow that can aid in creating a fire, but in damp, humid, or rainy weather, fire-starting becomes more challenging. To mitigate this, ancient survivalists would use natural shelters, like rock overhangs, to protect their efforts from rain and wind. Similarly, collecting dry tinder, often hidden within the bark or inner layers of plants, and using kindling that catches easily, such as twigs or dried moss, are essential strategies in challenging conditions. Building a fire in a cone shape or adding larger logs once the fire is established ensures that it stays burning without smothering the flame, reflecting an understanding of airflow and fuel needs.

The process of fire-starting without modern tools embodies an ancient relationship with nature, one that emphasizes patience, persistence, and a knowledge of the resources available. Mastery of these techniques takes time and practice, as each method requires specific materials, weather conditions, and physical skills. However, once learned, these methods offer a profound sense of resilience, connecting us to the survival strategies of our ancestors and reminding us of the essential role fire plays in human life. In many ways, fire-starting without tools is both a survival skill and a meditation on human ingenuity, resourcefulness, and our enduring bond with the natural world.

Navigating without a Compass: Using Sun, Stars, and Landmarks

Navigating without a compass, an ancient skill honed by explorers, traders, and survivalists, is a profound and essential part of self-sufficiency in wilderness settings. This skill harnesses the natural world—observing the sun, stars, and distinctive landmarks to establish direction and navigate across landscapes. Learning to read these environmental clues taps into thousands of years of human experience and provides an invaluable backup when technology fails. While the specific techniques vary according to climate and geography, each method offers reliable insights, empowering individuals to traverse unfamiliar terrain with confidence.

The sun is one of the most consistent and accessible tools for natural navigation. Because it rises roughly in the east and sets in the west, the sun's path provides a baseline for establishing direction. In the early morning, the sun appears low in the eastern sky, marking an approximate eastward direction. As the day progresses, the sun arcs through the sky, reaching its highest point in the south in the Northern Hemisphere and in the north in the Southern Hemisphere at midday. By late afternoon and evening, it descends in the western sky, indicating westward. This predictable motion can help establish an approximate east-west line, which in turn makes north-south orientation possible. For example, if you are facing the sunrise, your right side would roughly correspond to the south in the Northern Hemisphere and to the north in the Southern Hemisphere.

One of the most practical methods for navigating by the sun is the "shadow-stick" technique. This method involves placing a stick vertically in the ground, then observing the shadow it casts. Initially, the shadow points west. After about 15 to 30 minutes, the shadow will have moved slightly as the sun's position changes. Marking the initial and new positions of the shadow will create a line running roughly west to east, with the first shadow mark representing west and the second mark indicating east. Drawing a perpendicular line from the center of these points helps determine the north-south axis. This simple setup can be used even on cloudy days if enough sunlight filters through, providing a reliable orientation point for continued navigation.

Aside from direct observation, certain environmental indicators influenced by the sun's position can also guide direction. For instance, moss tends to grow on the more shaded, often northern, sides of trees in the Northern Hemisphere, as it prefers damp, less sunny locations. Likewise, snow typically melts more slowly on the north-facing slopes. These natural markers, however, can vary depending on factors like regional climate or local ecology. While not as precise as direct sun navigation, such clues can nonetheless offer helpful hints for orientation, particularly when used in conjunction with other methods.

As day turns to night, the stars become invaluable navigational aids. For millennia, people around the world have used star patterns to determine direction, taking advantage of the night sky's stability. The North Star, also known as Polaris, is the most well-known celestial marker for navigation in the Northern Hemisphere. Located almost directly above the North Pole, Polaris appears almost stationary in the night sky, making it a fixed point around which other stars rotate. To locate Polaris, one can use the Big Dipper constellation as a reference. The two stars forming the outer edge of the Big Dipper's "bowl" point directly toward Polaris, making it relatively easy to find. Once located, Polaris provides a reliable northward direction, simplifying orientation for those traveling north or wanting to establish a baseline direction.

In the Southern Hemisphere, the absence of a direct counterpart to Polaris necessitates a different approach. Instead of a single bright star, navigators use the Southern Cross constellation. The Southern Cross, shaped like a kite, includes four bright stars that form a cross-like shape in the sky. Drawing an imaginary line from the long axis of the cross downwards points roughly towards the South Pole. By extending this line to the horizon, one can estimate the southern direction, offering a functional guide for those journeying southward. Although not as precise as Polaris, the Southern Cross is still a valuable and dependable aid for finding direction at night.

In both hemispheres, other constellations and stars can provide secondary references to help maintain orientation. Orion, for instance, appears prominently in both Northern and Southern Hemisphere skies and rises in the east and sets in the west, providing a general sense of direction. The star Sirius, located below Orion's belt, is one of the brightest in the night sky and can serve as an additional point of reference. By becoming familiar with the night sky's prominent features, navigators can feel more confident finding their way even on overcast nights when only a few stars might be visible.

While the sun and stars offer direction in open terrain, landmarks play an equally important role in natural navigation, especially in forests, mountains, and other densely vegetated environments. Mountains, rivers, distinctive tree formations, and even unusual rock outcroppings serve as reference points that can help create a mental map of the surroundings. In ancient navigation, these landmarks were integral, as travelers memorized specific routes by marking prominent features along their journey. Even subtle features, such as the shape of a ridgeline or a particular bend in a river, can guide direction and serve as orientation aids.

Navigating by river flow is one useful strategy, especially when in unknown areas. Most rivers flow consistently toward larger bodies of water, such as lakes, seas, or oceans. By following a river downstream, one can often reach populated areas or points of interest, which can provide an additional layer of safety in survival situations. Moreover, river valleys tend to cut through landscapes, offering easier paths compared to hilly or mountainous areas.

Observing the river's flow, direction, and associated flora can also provide clues about the environment, enhancing one's sense of direction and awareness of the natural world.

Another landmark-based navigation method involves understanding the local wind patterns, which can sometimes remain consistent, especially in coastal regions. For instance, along shorelines, daytime sea breezes often blow inland, while night breezes reverse direction. Understanding these patterns, which are influenced by the daily heating and cooling of land and water, can help confirm a navigational path, particularly in open areas where other landmarks may be sparse. Observing tree growth, which can sometimes lean in the direction of prevailing winds, can also offer a subtle clue about direction, though this method is less reliable in areas with irregular wind patterns.

The use of animal behavior, though an unconventional navigational tool, can also provide subtle hints about direction. Birds, for example, typically fly toward water sources at dawn and dusk, while insects like ants often establish trails leading to consistent food sources, which can sometimes correlate with nearby water or vegetation. Paying attention to animal trails, especially those leading downhill, may guide toward water sources or lower altitudes. Though these clues require close observation, they can add valuable insight into orientation and terrain layout.

Ultimately, navigating without a compass demands patience, observation, and an awareness of the environment. By combining various techniques—observing the sun's path, recognizing star patterns, and noting landmarks—one can piece together a comprehensive understanding of direction. This reliance on natural cues fosters a sense of connection with the land and sharpens one's instincts, providing a reliable approach to finding one's way in any environment. Although each method may present challenges, mastery of these ancient navigation techniques can make travel through unknown terrains manageable, and, in some cases, even enjoyable, as each journey becomes an exercise in understanding and working with nature's subtle guidance.

Foraging for Food and Medicinal Plants

Foraging for edible wild plants and herbs is an ancient practice that has sustained human populations across various cultures and climates. This skill connects us deeply to the natural world, offering not only a source of nutrition but also a profound understanding of local ecosystems. With the ability to identify and harvest wild plants, individuals can enhance their self-sufficiency and survival skills, supplementing diets with fresh, nutrient-rich foods. However, foraging requires knowledge, respect for the environment, and caution, as not all wild plants are safe for consumption.

Edible wild plants fall into several categories, including greens, roots, seeds, nuts, fruits, and herbs. Each category contributes uniquely to a forager's diet, providing essential vitamins, minerals, and flavors that can enhance meals. Wild greens, such as dandelion, nettle, and lamb's quarters, are among the most common edible plants found in diverse environments. Dandelion, for example, is often dismissed as a mere weed, yet its leaves are rich in vitamins A, C, and K, as well as minerals like iron and calcium. The young leaves can be harvested in spring for salads, while the roots can be dried and roasted as a coffee substitute.

Nettle, another nutritious green, is often overlooked due to its stinging hairs. However, once cooked, the stinging properties diminish, revealing a flavor reminiscent of spinach. Nettles are high in vitamins A and C, iron, and calcium, making them a valuable addition to soups, stews, and teas. The leaves can be harvested in early spring, and careful handling with gloves during collection ensures a safe foraging experience. Lamb's quarters, often found in gardens and disturbed soils, are similarly nutritious, boasting a flavor akin to spinach and providing substantial amounts of vitamin A, vitamin C, and calcium. The leaves can be enjoyed raw in salads or cooked like other leafy greens.

Roots and tubers also represent a vital component of wild foraging. Plants like wild garlic, wild onion, and various types of wild carrots can provide hearty and flavorful additions to meals. Wild garlic and onion, both members of the Allium family, are often found in woodlands and can be identified by their distinct aroma. The bulbs and leaves are edible and can be used to flavor dishes or consumed raw in salads. Wild carrots, such as Queen Anne's lace, can be recognized by their lacy flowers and feathery leaves. However, caution is essential, as some similar-looking plants, such as poison hemlock, are toxic. Proper identification is crucial, and foragers should consult reliable guides or experts before consuming unfamiliar plants.

Seeds and nuts also offer nutritional benefits, particularly as sources of healthy fats and proteins. Acorns, for example, are a traditional food source for many indigenous cultures. However, they require processing to remove tannins, which can cause bitterness. The acorns can be leached in water to remove these compounds before being ground into flour or used in various recipes. Other nut-bearing trees, such as chestnuts and hickories, can be foraged for their edible nuts, which are delicious when roasted and provide a rich source of energy.

Fruits and berries represent another essential category of edible wild plants. Depending on the season, foragers may find a variety of wild fruits, including blackberries, raspberries, blueberries, and elderberries. Wild fruits not only offer sweetness and flavor but also provide vitamins, antioxidants, and dietary fiber. Elderberries, for instance, are rich in vitamins A and C and are commonly used in syrups, jams. However, it's vital to cook elderberries before consumption, as raw berries can cause digestive discomfort. Wild strawberries, a favorite among foragers, are small but packed with flavor, making them perfect for snacking or incorporating into desserts.

Herbs also play a significant role in foraging, as they can enhance flavors and provide medicinal benefits. Common edible herbs include wild mint, wild thyme, and yarrow. Wild mint, often found near water sources, can be used in teas, desserts, or as a seasoning for savory dishes. Its aromatic leaves add a refreshing flavor to salads and drinks. Wild thyme, recognizable by its small purple flowers and trailing habit, can also be used in various culinary applications, bringing a fragrant herbaceous note to dishes. Yarrow, on the other hand, is primarily valued for its medicinal properties. Traditionally used to stop bleeding and reduce inflammation, yarrow can be made into teas or poultices for various ailments.

Foraging requires careful attention to the environment and ethical considerations. It is essential to respect local ecosystems by foraging sustainably and responsibly. When harvesting wild plants, foragers should take care not to deplete local populations, leaving enough for wildlife and ensuring plants can regenerate. A good rule of thumb is to harvest no more than one-third of a plant or a specific area, allowing for future growth and minimizing ecological impact. Foragers should also be mindful of the laws and regulations regarding wild plant harvesting in their area, as some locations may restrict or prohibit foraging to protect native species and habitats.

Proper identification of plants is crucial to successful foraging. Many edible plants have toxic look-alikes that can cause illness or even be fatal if consumed. To avoid confusion, foragers should invest time in learning about the specific plants they wish to harvest. Field guides, foraging workshops, and mentorship from experienced foragers can provide valuable insights and practical knowledge. Observing the habitat, growth patterns, and distinctive features of plants will help build a forager's confidence in identifying edible species.

In addition to nutrition, many wild plants offer medicinal properties that have been recognized by traditional healing practices. For instance, dandelion is not only edible but also serves as a natural diuretic and digestive aid. Similarly, plantain leaves can be used to soothe insect bites and skin irritations, while chamomile can be harvested for its calming tea. This dual-purpose aspect of foraging highlights the interconnectedness of food and medicine, reinforcing the idea that many wild plants have long been integral to human survival.

Finally, learning to forage for wild plants fosters a deep connection to the land and a sense of appreciation for the natural world. It encourages individuals to observe their surroundings more closely, understanding the seasonal rhythms of nature and the resources available within their local ecosystems. As foragers develop their skills and knowledge, they cultivate a profound respect for the environment, recognizing the importance of biodiversity and the value of maintaining a healthy ecosystem.

In conclusion, foraging for edible wild plants and herbs is a time-honored practice that enriches both diet and well-being. By harnessing the knowledge of local flora, individuals can enhance their self-sufficiency while fostering a deeper connection to nature. With careful observation, proper identification, and sustainable practices, foraging provides not only sustenance but also a valuable opportunity to engage with the natural world in meaningful ways. As more people turn to foraging, this ancient skill continues to weave itself into contemporary life, bridging the gap between our ancestral roots and the modern quest for self-sufficiency and connection to the earth.

Recognizing and Avoiding Poisonous Plants

Foraging for wild plants can be a rewarding endeavor, providing fresh food and herbal remedies; however, the knowledge of how to recognize and avoid poisonous plants is crucial for ensuring safety in the wild. Throughout history, humans have developed an intimate understanding of their local flora, learning which plants are edible and which can be toxic. This knowledge is essential, as many poisonous plants closely resemble their edible counterparts, making identification challenging. Familiarity with specific characteristics, habitat preferences, and key species is vital for anyone venturing into the world of foraging.

Poisonous plants can be broadly categorized into three types: those that cause mild gastrointestinal distress, those that can lead to severe illness or death, and those that result in skin irritation. Understanding the effects of these plants and being able to identify them can help foragers avoid potential dangers. Mildly toxic plants may cause symptoms such as nausea, vomiting, or diarrhea but are unlikely to cause long-term harm. In contrast, some plants contain compounds that can lead to severe health issues or even death, often affecting the liver, kidneys, or nervous system. Skin irritants, while not necessarily life-threatening, can cause painful reactions upon contact and should also be avoided.

One of the most critical aspects of recognizing poisonous plants is learning to identify their unique features. Many toxic plants have distinctive characteristics that set them apart from their edible relatives. For instance, the infamous poison hemlock (Conium maculatum) is often confused with edible wild carrots or parsley. However, poison hemlock can be distinguished by its smooth, hairless stems that are marked with purple spots and its fern-like leaves. The flowers of poison hemlock grow in umbrella-like clusters, similar to those of the carrot family, but they tend to be small and white.

Another notorious plant is the deadly nightshade (Atropa belladonna), which bears shiny black berries and bell-shaped purple flowers. While its berries may seem enticing, they contain potent alkaloids that can lead to severe poisoning or death if consumed. In contrast, edible plants such as blueberries or huckleberries, which have similar-looking berries, are entirely safe. Familiarizing oneself with the characteristics of these plants and their growing conditions can help prevent dangerous mistakes.

Common poison ivy (Toxicodendron radicans), poison oak (Toxicodendron diversilobum), and poison sumac (Toxicodendron vernix) are examples of skin irritants that foragers should be wary of when exploring natural areas. These plants contain an oil called urushiol, which can trigger severe allergic reactions in sensitive individuals. Poison ivy is easily recognized by its characteristic "leaves of three," while poison oak has similarly lobed leaves that resemble oak leaves. Poison sumac, which prefers wet habitats, can be identified by its clusters of yellow-green berries and compound leaves with up to 13 leaflets. Avoiding contact with these plants is essential, as even a small amount of urushiol can cause a painful rash and significant discomfort.

In addition to visual identification, understanding the habitat preferences of poisonous plants can aid in avoidance. Many toxic plants thrive in specific environments, so knowing where to look can help foragers stay safe. For example, poison ivy is often found in wooded areas, along trails, and in gardens, while poison hemlock prefers wet, disturbed soils near roadsides or streams. By familiarizing oneself with the environments where these plants grow, foragers can better navigate their surroundings and reduce the risk of encountering hazardous flora.

While visual identification is vital, it is equally important to learn the characteristics of edible plants that could be confused with poisonous varieties. Developing a mental library of images, descriptions, and habitats of common edible plants can help foragers make informed decisions while out in the field. For instance, learning to distinguish between wild garlic (Allium vineale) and its toxic look-alike, which is often mistaken for a wild onion, can prevent mishaps. Wild garlic can be recognized by its distinct garlic odor, while the toxic plant lacks this characteristic scent.

To further ensure safety while foraging, some practical tips can help avoid the risks associated with poisonous plants. First, always carry a reliable field guide or app that provides clear images and descriptions of both edible and poisonous plants. This can be an invaluable resource for cross-referencing and confirming identifications in the field. Additionally, when foraging with others, sharing knowledge and observations can provide an extra layer of safety, as multiple sets of eyes can help identify potential hazards.

Another important rule is to avoid consuming any wild plant unless you can positively identify it. Even if a plant is traditionally deemed edible, variations and look-alikes can lead to confusion. If uncertain about a plant's safety, it is always best to err on the side of caution and refrain from consumption. Many foragers follow the "test small" rule, which suggests trying a small quantity of a new plant first, waiting to see if any adverse reactions occur before consuming larger amounts. However, this approach should only be used with plants that are known to be edible and whose toxic counterparts have been confidently identified.

Education and experience are crucial to successful foraging. Joining foraging groups or attending workshops led by knowledgeable foragers can provide hands-on learning opportunities and foster a deeper understanding of plant identification. Additionally, local conservation organizations or botanical gardens often offer guided foraging tours, which can help individuals learn about native plants and their uses in a safe environment.

In conclusion, recognizing and avoiding poisonous plants is an essential skill for anyone interested in foraging for food and medicinal plants. By developing a keen eye for identifying toxic species and understanding their habitats, foragers can minimize risks and enjoy the benefits of wild harvesting. Educating oneself through field guides, workshops, and experience is crucial to building confidence and expertise in this ancient practice. The world of foraging is rich with rewards, but it requires respect, caution, and a commitment to learning. By fostering a connection with the natural world and prioritizing safety, individuals can safely explore the abundant resources that wild plants offer while avoiding the dangers that accompany them.

Ancient Foraging Techniques and Seasonal Harvesting

Foraging is not merely a practice; it is an age-old tradition rooted in the fundamental relationship between humans and nature. Ancient foragers honed techniques that allowed them to thrive in their environments, adapting to the rhythms of nature and the changing seasons. These practices, passed down through generations, provide invaluable lessons in sustainability, self-sufficiency, and respect for the earth. Understanding ancient foraging techniques and seasonal harvesting enables modern foragers to connect with their ancestral roots while cultivating a deeper appreciation for the bounty that nature provides.

At the heart of ancient foraging was an intimate knowledge of the landscape and its seasonal cycles. Early humans relied on keen observation to identify when specific plants were at their peak ripeness, ensuring optimal nutrition and flavor. This understanding of seasonal changes was essential for survival, as it dictated the availability of food sources throughout the year. For instance, in temperate regions, spring heralded the emergence of tender greens and shoots, while summer brought forth an abundance of fruits and seeds. Autumn signaled the time to harvest nuts and roots, and winter often required foragers to rely on preserved foods or foraging for hardy greens that could withstand the frost.

One of the most significant aspects of ancient foraging techniques was the use of knowledge accumulated over generations. Indigenous peoples and early agricultural societies developed extensive ethnobotanical knowledge, understanding which plants were edible, medicinal, or toxic. This wisdom was often shared through oral traditions, storytelling, and hands-on experience. The seasonal calendar was an essential tool, as it allowed foragers to track the cyclical nature of plant growth and animal behavior. For example, certain plants, like wild garlic and spring beauty, are best harvested in early spring when their nutrient content is highest, while others, such as elderberries and blackberries, are best collected in late summer.

In addition to seasonal knowledge, ancient foragers employed various techniques to maximize their harvests. One common method was to use specific tools crafted from natural materials. Simple implements made from stone, bone, or wood enabled foragers to dig, scrape, and gather edible plants with efficiency. For instance, digging sticks made from sturdy branches or sharpened stones were used to unearth tubers and roots, while baskets woven from flexible grasses or reeds were utilized for gathering fruits and berries. These tools not only facilitated the harvesting process but also exemplified the resourcefulness of ancient peoples in adapting to their environments.

Another vital technique was the practice of polyculture foraging, where multiple plants were harvested from the same area. Ancient foragers understood the benefits of biodiversity and often sought out areas where different species grew in proximity. This approach not only ensured a varied diet but also helped maintain the health of the ecosystem. By harvesting different plants at different times, foragers contributed to the regeneration of the land, as some plants thrived in the wake of others being removed. This cyclical approach to foraging is a cornerstone of sustainable practices, demonstrating an intrinsic respect for the balance of nature.

Seasonal harvesting also involved an awareness of animal behavior and ecology. Ancient foragers knew that certain animals would emerge or migrate with the changing seasons, providing opportunities for hunting and gathering. For example, the return of migratory birds in spring signaled the time to hunt for protein-rich foods, while the seasonal movement of game animals, such as deer, dictated when and where to set traps or plan hunts. This interconnectedness of plants and animals in the ecosystem was crucial for survival, and ancient foragers were adept at reading the signs of nature to optimize their harvesting strategies.

Additionally, traditional knowledge encompassed techniques for preserving food for the off-season. Ancient peoples employed methods such as drying, smoking, and fermenting to extend the shelf life of perishable items. For instance, berries could be dried in the sun or smoked to create nutritious snacks for winter months. Roots and tubers were often stored in cool, dark places or submerged in water to maintain their freshness. Fermentation was used to preserve seasonal harvests, transforming fruits into beverages or vegetables into pickled delights. This ingenuity ensured that communities could endure through harsh winters when fresh food sources were scarce.

The practice of foraging also carried with it a spiritual and cultural significance. Many ancient societies revered the natural world and its resources, integrating foraging into their cultural practices and beliefs. Seasonal festivals often celebrated the harvest, reinforcing the connection between humans and the earth. Rituals surrounding the gathering of specific plants or the first fruits of the season fostered a sense of gratitude and respect for the resources that sustained them. This cultural connection to foraging not only shaped their diets but also their identities, as communities came together to share knowledge, stories, and experiences related to the land.

In contemporary society, there is a growing recognition of the importance of these ancient foraging techniques. As people seek to reconnect with nature and embrace self-sufficiency, the wisdom of our ancestors offers valuable insights. Modern foragers can learn from traditional practices, adapting them to current environments while remaining mindful of sustainability. By understanding the seasonal patterns of local flora and fauna, individuals can cultivate a deeper relationship with their surroundings, fostering a sense of stewardship for the land.

In conclusion, ancient foraging techniques and seasonal harvesting are fundamental aspects of humanity's relationship with nature. The wisdom of our ancestors, rooted in observation, respect, and resourcefulness, continues to inform modern foraging practices. By embracing these techniques and honoring the rhythms of the natural world, individuals can cultivate self-sufficiency, deepen their connection to the environment, and honor the traditions of those who came before us. As we navigate the challenges of contemporary life, the lessons learned from ancient foragers serve as a guiding light, reminding us of the enduring bond between humans and the earth's abundant resources.

The art of food preservation is a time-honored practice that has sustained human societies for millennia. In ancient times, the necessity of extending the shelf life of seasonal produce was crucial for survival, especially during harsh winters or times of scarcity. Long before the advent of refrigeration and modern canning techniques, our ancestors developed various natural methods for preserving food, ensuring they had access to nourishment throughout the year. Understanding these ancient techniques not only connects us with our culinary heritage but also empowers us to utilize sustainable practices in our contemporary kitchens.

The fundamental principles of natural food preservation revolve around inhibiting the growth of microorganisms, slowing down enzymatic processes, and minimizing exposure to air and light. Various methods, including drying, fermenting, pickling, and cold storage, harness the power of nature to enhance the longevity of food. Each method carries its unique techniques, advantages, and flavor profiles, allowing for a diverse array of preserved foods that contribute to a well-rounded diet.

One of the oldest and most straightforward methods of food preservation is drying. This technique involves removing moisture from fruits, vegetables, herbs, and meats, as water is essential for the growth of bacteria, yeasts, and molds. Ancient cultures utilized the sun's natural heat to dehydrate foods, laying sliced fruits and vegetables on flat surfaces or hanging them from lines. Sun-dried tomatoes, apricots, and herbs are just a few examples of the delightful products of this method.

In cooler climates or during seasons when sunlight is scarce, ancient peoples relied on wind and airflow for drying. They constructed drying racks or used smokehouses, which combined drying and smoking, to preserve meats and fish. The process of smoking not only dehydrates the food but also infuses it with unique flavors while providing an additional layer of protection against spoilage. Smoked salmon and jerky are contemporary representations of these ancient preservation techniques, demonstrating how they remain relevant and effective today.

Fermentation is another powerful method of preservation that ancient cultures embraced for both its practicality and health benefits. This process relies on the natural activity of beneficial bacteria and yeasts to convert sugars into acids, gases, creating an inhospitable environment for harmful microorganisms. Fermented foods such as sauerkraut, kimchi, yogurt, and pickles not only have extended shelf lives but also offer probiotics, which support gut health and enhance digestion.

The fermentation process begins with the selection of fresh, high-quality produce. For vegetables, such as cabbage for sauerkraut or cucumbers for pickling, the natural sugars present provide the food source for beneficial microorganisms. Salt is often added to create a brine, which helps draw out moisture and create an anaerobic environment necessary for fermentation. This brine not only flavors the vegetables but also prevents spoilage. Over a few weeks, the fermentation process transforms the vegetables, resulting in tangy, flavorful foods that can last for months or even years when stored properly.

Another traditional preservation method is pickling, which involves submerging foods in an acidic solution, typically vinegar or brine. This technique was widely used in ancient cultures to prolong the life of vegetables, fruits, and even fish. The high acidity of the pickling solution inhibits bacterial growth while imparting bold flavors. Classic examples of pickled foods include dill pickles, pickled onions, and pickled beets. Ancient civilizations often combined spices, herbs, and other flavorings to create distinctive pickles that reflected local culinary traditions.

Cold storage is a preservation method that relies on low temperatures to slow down the deterioration of food. While modern refrigeration has made this technique commonplace, ancient peoples employed various forms of cold storage long before electric appliances existed. In colder climates, root cellars were dug into the earth to maintain a consistent cool temperature, protecting vegetables like carrots, potatoes, and turnips from freezing while ensuring they remained fresh. This natural cooling method extended the shelf life of seasonal harvests, allowing families to enjoy the fruits of their labor well into the winter months.

In warmer regions, ancient peoples discovered that burying food in cool, damp earth could extend its life. Techniques varied by culture, but methods such as wrapping food in leaves and placing it in a cool stream or burying it in the ground with moist soil were common. This approach not only preserved the food but also offered unique flavors through natural fermentation processes that occurred underground.

Another natural method that has stood the test of time is salting. Salting meats and fish draws out moisture, creating a hostile environment for bacteria.

Ancient cultures utilized salt as a preservation method for centuries, particularly in coastal areas where fish were abundant. Salted fish, such as cod or herring, could be stored for long periods, making it a valuable protein source during lean times. The technique of curing meats with salt, spices, and sugar has also produced beloved delicacies, such as prosciutto and smoked bacon.

While these ancient techniques are incredibly effective, they require careful attention to hygiene and conditions to prevent spoilage. Ensuring that equipment, containers, and ingredients are clean is essential for success in any preservation method. Using glass jars, ceramic crocks, or food-grade containers can help maintain the integrity of preserved foods. Moreover, labeling and dating preserved items can prevent confusion and ensure that older products are used first, minimizing waste.

As we rediscover these ancient preservation methods, it is vital to understand their cultural significance and the deep respect for the land and resources they embody. Each technique is a reflection of the natural environment, local ingredients, and the ingenuity of the people who practiced them. By adopting these natural preservation methods, we not only enhance our culinary experiences but also honor the traditions and wisdom of our ancestors.

In conclusion, preserving food naturally for long-term storage is a practice that has sustained humanity for generations. The techniques of drying, fermenting, pickling, cold storage, and salting are all time-tested methods that allow us to enjoy seasonal bounty throughout the year. By reconnecting with these ancient practices, we can cultivate self-sufficiency, reduce waste, and appreciate the flavors and nutrition that preserved foods offer. Embracing these techniques not only enhances our culinary skills but also fosters a deeper relationship with the land and its resources, reminding us of the enduring connection between humans and nature.

Ancient Methods of Food Preservation

Food preservation has been a cornerstone of human survival, allowing societies to extend the shelf life of their food supplies and ensure nourishment during times of scarcity. Among the myriad techniques developed over millennia, fermentation, drying, and smoking stand out as particularly effective and culturally significant methods. These ancient practices not only helped prevent spoilage but also transformed food into diverse and flavorful forms, enriching the human diet and preserving cultural heritage.

Fermentation is a natural process that relies on the activity of microorganisms—yeasts and bacteria—to convert sugars and starches into acids, gases. This method has been utilized by various cultures around the world for centuries, creating a plethora of food and beverage options that are both delicious and nutritious. The science behind fermentation hinges on creating an anaerobic environment, which inhibits harmful bacteria while promoting the growth of beneficial microbes.

One of the most familiar fermented foods is yogurt, which originated in the Middle East and Central Asia. The process begins with milk, which is heated and then cooled to a specific temperature. Once at the right temperature, live bacterial cultures are introduced, typically Lactobacillus bulgaricus and Streptococcus thermophilus. These bacteria ferment the lactose in the milk, producing lactic acid, which thickens the milk and gives yogurt its characteristic tangy flavor. This simple process not only preserves the milk but also enhances its nutritional profile by increasing digestibility and providing probiotics that support gut health.

Sauerkraut, a fermented cabbage dish, is another excellent example of this ancient technique. The process of making sauerkraut begins with shredding fresh cabbage and mixing it with salt. The salt draws out moisture from the cabbage, creating a brine in which the natural fermentation can occur. Over a few weeks, lactic acid bacteria convert the sugars in the cabbage into lactic acid, resulting in a crunchy, tangy condiment that can be stored for months. This process not only preserves the cabbage but also imparts unique flavors and nutritional benefits, making sauerkraut a staple in many cuisines.

Kimchi, a traditional Korean dish, exemplifies the variety and complexity of fermentation. Made primarily from Napa cabbage and radishes, kimchi is seasoned with chili pepper, garlic, ginger, and other spices. The mixture is then salted and allowed to ferment in jars. This process can vary from a few days to several weeks, depending on the desired flavor and fermentation level. Kimchi is rich in vitamins, probiotics, and antioxidants, showcasing how fermentation can enhance both flavor and health benefits.

Drying is one of the oldest methods of food preservation, dating back thousands of years. The primary principle behind drying is to remove moisture from food, which inhibits the growth of bacteria, yeasts, and molds. Ancient peoples utilized the sun's heat to dehydrate fruits, vegetables, herbs, and meats, creating a variety of preserved foods that could be stored for extended periods. Sun-drying was common in many cultures, especially in arid regions where the sun was strong and temperatures were high.

Fruits such as figs, dates, and apricots were often sun-dried to concentrate their flavors and extend their shelf life. This method was especially crucial in ancient societies, where the harvest season was limited. Dried fruits provided essential nutrients and energy during times of scarcity, making them a vital component of the diet. Additionally, dried fruits were often used in cooking and baking, adding sweetness and texture to dishes.

Vegetables were also commonly dried, with techniques varying across cultures. In Mediterranean regions, tomatoes were often sliced and sun-dried, resulting in a concentrated flavor that could be used in sauces, stews, and salads. In Asia, various vegetables, including mushrooms, peppers, and green beans, were dehydrated for preservation and later rehydrated for use in soups and stir-fries.

The drying of meats, known as jerky, is another ancient preservation method that allowed nomadic cultures to transport protein sources over long distances. By salting and drying meat, such as beef or fish, ancient peoples could create nutrient-dense food that was lightweight and had a long shelf life. The technique not only prevented spoilage but also added unique flavors, as the drying process intensified the natural taste of the meat.

Smoking combines drying with the addition of flavor, offering yet another effective preservation method. Ancient cultures discovered that exposing food to smoke from burning wood could inhibit bacterial growth while imparting distinctive flavors. Smoking has been used for centuries to preserve meats and fish, particularly in coastal areas where seafood was abundant.

The smoking process typically involves curing the meat or fish with salt before exposing it to smoke. The smoke contains phenols and other compounds that create a protective barrier against spoilage while infusing the food with rich flavors. Common examples of smoked foods include salmon, trout, and various cuts of meat, such as ham and bacon. Each type of wood used in the smoking process imparts its unique flavor profile, creating a wide range of culinary possibilities.

In addition to enhancing flavor, smoking also plays a significant role in food preservation. The low temperatures and high humidity levels during the smoking process help to remove moisture from the food, further extending its shelf life. This technique was especially important for communities living in remote areas or regions where access to fresh food was limited.

The cultural significance of fermentation, drying, and smoking extends beyond mere food preservation. These methods are often deeply embedded in the culinary traditions and social practices of various cultures. For example, the making of kimchi is often a communal activity in Korean households, with families coming together to prepare large batches for the winter months. Similarly, smoking meats and fish has been a ritualistic practice in many Indigenous cultures, celebrating the connection between food, nature, and community.

In contemporary society, there is a renewed interest in these ancient preservation methods as people seek sustainable and natural ways to store food. The resurgence of interest in fermentation has led to a boom in the production of artisanal foods such as craft beers, kombucha, and probiotic-rich foods. Home cooks are increasingly experimenting with these techniques, preserving seasonal harvests and creating unique flavors in their kitchens.

As we delve into the world of food preservation through fermentation, drying, and smoking, we are not only connecting with our culinary heritage but also embracing a sustainable lifestyle. These ancient methods remind us of the importance of utilizing local resources, minimizing waste, and fostering a deeper relationship with the food we consume. By understanding and practicing these techniques, we can ensure that the flavors and nutritional benefits of our harvests are preserved for future generations to enjoy.

In conclusion, fermentation, drying, and smoking are foundational techniques in the ancient practice of food preservation. Each method offers unique benefits, flavors, and cultural significance, highlighting the ingenuity of our ancestors in ensuring their survival. As we embrace these time-honored practices in our modern kitchens, we not only enrich our diets but also honor the traditions and wisdom passed down through generations. Whether through tangy fermented vegetables, sun-dried fruits, or smoky meats, these ancient methods of preservation continue to play a vital role in our culinary landscape, connecting us to the past while guiding us toward a more sustainable future.

Storing Grains, Nuts, and Seeds for the Long Haul

The preservation of grains, nuts, and seeds is a fundamental aspect of ancient survival strategies that has persisted through the ages. These staple foods provide essential nutrients, energy, and versatility in various culinary applications. Proper storage techniques are crucial for extending the shelf life of these items, protecting them from pests, moisture, and spoilage, and ensuring that they remain a reliable food source over time. Understanding the methods our ancestors used to store these vital resources not only pays homage to their ingenuity but also equips us with the knowledge to sustain ourselves today.

Grains, such as wheat, rice, corn, and barley, have been staples of human diets for thousands of years. Their preservation has played a pivotal role in agricultural societies, where harvests were often seasonal and food scarcity loomed large. Ancient peoples developed various storage techniques to protect grains from environmental factors and pests, enabling them to store surplus harvests for future consumption.

One of the earliest methods of grain storage involved using underground pits. These pits provided a cool and dark environment that helped maintain a stable temperature and humidity level, crucial for preserving the quality of the grains. To create a grain pit, ancient farmers would dig a hole in the ground and line it with straw, leaves, or other natural materials to absorb moisture and prevent spoilage. Once the grains were placed inside, the pit was covered with more straw and earth to keep out pests and protect the grains from the elements.

In addition to underground pits, ancient cultures also employed clay or ceramic containers to store grains. These containers were often sealed with lids to keep out moisture and air, which could lead to spoilage. Clay jars were used by civilizations such as the Egyptians and Mesopotamians, who understood the importance of airtight storage. These containers were often placed in cool, dry places to minimize exposure to heat and humidity.

In more temperate climates, wooden granaries or elevated storage structures were constructed to protect grains from rodents and insects. These granaries allowed for airflow, reducing the risk of moisture accumulation and promoting longer shelf life. The use of slatted wooden floors prevented direct contact between the stored grains and the ground, further deterring pests. This method showcased the ingenuity of ancient builders in creating structures that addressed both storage needs and pest control.

The preservation of nuts and seeds, while somewhat similar to grains, requires attention to their unique characteristics. Nuts, such as almonds, walnuts, and hazelnuts, contain healthy oils that can turn rancid if not stored correctly. Ancient peoples often utilized natural methods to keep nuts fresh for extended periods. One common technique involved storing nuts in their shells, which acted as a protective barrier against environmental factors. By keeping the nuts in their shells, the risk of spoilage was significantly reduced, as the shells helped shield the delicate nuts from light, moisture, and pests.

For long-term storage, nuts were often buried in the ground or placed in cool, dark locations. Some cultures even used leaves, straw, or sand to further insulate the nuts from temperature fluctuations. The ancient Greeks, for instance, used to bury their walnuts in the ground to keep them fresh. In addition to burying, some societies would also immerse nuts in water or oil to prevent rancidity, a technique that continues to be employed in various culinary traditions today.

Seeds, like grains and nuts, require specific storage conditions to maintain their viability. Ancient farmers understood the importance of preserving seeds for future planting seasons. To ensure seeds remained viable for years, they were often dried thoroughly before storage. Drying seeds removes moisture, preventing fungal growth and decay.

Once dried, seeds were commonly stored in clay pots or woven baskets, similar to grains. The containers were kept in dark, cool places to minimize exposure to light and temperature fluctuations. In some cultures, seeds were wrapped in cloth or leaves to provide an additional layer of protection. This attention to detail reflected the understanding that seed viability depended on maintaining optimal storage conditions.

Today, modern techniques for storing grains, nuts, and seeds build upon these ancient methods while utilizing advancements in technology. Vacuum sealing, for instance, has become a popular option for long-term storage. By removing air from packaging, vacuum sealing prevents oxidation and spoilage, ensuring that these foods maintain their freshness and nutritional value. Additionally, modern refrigeration can significantly extend the shelf life of nuts and seeds, providing an effective way to keep their oils from going rancid.

Despite these advancements, the fundamental principles of food storage established by ancient civilizations remain relevant. Understanding the importance of cool, dark, and dry conditions is crucial for preserving the integrity of grains, nuts, and seeds. Regularly checking stored foods for signs of spoilage or pest infestations is also essential to maintaining their quality over time.

Moreover, the concept of batch rotation, a practice rooted in ancient agriculture, is vital for effective food storage. This practice involves using older stored foods first to prevent waste and ensure that nothing goes unused.

By implementing a first-in, first-out (FIFO) system, individuals can maintain a constant supply of fresh grains, nuts, and seeds while minimizing spoilage.

As we embrace these ancient methods of storing grains, nuts, and seeds, we also cultivate a deeper appreciation for the knowledge passed down through generations. These techniques reflect not only a survival strategy but also a profound connection to the earth and the resources it provides. By learning from our ancestors, we can continue to sustain ourselves and future generations, honoring their wisdom while adapting their practices to our modern lives.

In conclusion, the preservation of grains, nuts, and seeds is a critical aspect of ancient survival techniques that has endured through time. The use of underground pits, clay containers, granaries, and natural barriers illustrates the ingenuity of our ancestors in safeguarding these essential food sources. By understanding and adopting these methods, we can ensure that our grains, nuts, and seeds remain viable and nutritious for the long haul. Embracing these ancient practices not only enhances our self-sufficiency but also fosters a connection to the rich history of food preservation, allowing us to appreciate the enduring relationship between humans and the natural world.

Salt Preservation: Meat, Fish, and Vegetables

Salt preservation is one of the oldest and most effective methods for extending the shelf life of food, particularly meats, fish, and vegetables. This ancient technique leverages salt's natural ability to inhibit microbial growth, preventing spoilage and enabling people to store food for extended periods. The use of salt in preservation has been vital for civilizations throughout history, transforming the way food is stored and consumed. Understanding the principles behind salt preservation not only highlights its significance in ancient survival strategies but also provides valuable insights for modern food preservation practices.

The process of salt preservation, known as curing, involves the application of salt to food in various forms, either by dry salting or brining. This method works by drawing moisture out of the food through osmosis, creating an environment that is inhospitable to bacteria and fungi. As moisture is removed, salt penetrates the food, altering its structure and flavor while preserving its nutritional value.

Meat preservation through salting has been a cornerstone of culinary traditions worldwide. In ancient times, before refrigeration was available, curing meats was essential for survival. Different cultures developed unique curing techniques based on regional resources and preferences. One of the most common methods is dry curing, where salt is applied directly to the meat's surface. The meat is often coated in a generous layer of salt and allowed to rest for a specific period, during which the salt draws out moisture and flavors the meat.

One well-known example of dry curing is prosciutto, a traditional Italian ham. The process begins with selecting high-quality pork legs, which are then salted and left to cure for several months. The salt not only preserves the meat but also imparts a rich flavor and distinctive texture. Once cured, prosciutto can be sliced thin and served as a delicacy, showcasing the art of salt preservation.

Brining, another method of salt preservation, involves soaking meat in a saltwater solution. This technique is particularly effective for larger cuts of meat, as it ensures even salting throughout. The brine can also include sugar, spices, and herbs, adding depth of flavor to the final product. A classic example of this method is the preparation of corned beef, where beef brisket is brined with a mixture of salt, sugar, and pickling spices, resulting in a flavorful and tender meat that can be enjoyed in various dishes.

Fish preservation using salt is similarly ancient and vital for societies reliant on fishing. One of the earliest methods of preserving fish was salting, a technique that allowed communities to store their catch for months or even years. The practice of salting fish involves either dry salting or brining, depending on the desired outcome.

Dry salting fish is a straightforward process. Fresh fish are cleaned and gutted before being coated in salt. The salt draws out moisture, and the fish is left to cure for several hours or days, depending on the thickness of the fillets. This method creates a firm texture and concentrated flavor, ideal for dishes like salted cod, which has been a staple in many cultures. Salted cod is often rehydrated before cooking, allowing it to regain some moisture while retaining its characteristic taste.

Brining is another popular method for preserving fish. Similar to meat, fish can be soaked in a saltwater solution, sometimes combined with sugar and spices. This technique not only preserves the fish but also infuses it with additional flavors. One notable example is gravlax, a Nordic dish made by curing salmon with a mixture of salt, sugar, and dill. The result is a silky, flavorful fish that can be enjoyed raw or lightly smoked.

Vegetable preservation with salt has also played a crucial role in food storage. Salting vegetables helps draw out moisture, preventing spoilage and allowing them to be stored for extended periods. One of the oldest forms of vegetable preservation is pickling, which often involves using salt as a primary ingredient. In pickling, vegetables are submerged in a brine solution, which can include vinegar, salt, and spices.

The process of fermenting vegetables through salting has been practiced for centuries. Sauerkraut, for instance, is made by finely shredding cabbage and mixing it with salt. As the salt draws out moisture from the cabbage, lactic acid bacteria begin to ferment the sugars, resulting in a tangy, crunchy condiment. This method not only preserves the cabbage but also enriches it with probiotics, contributing to gut health.

Another example of salt preservation in vegetables is the preparation of salted cucumbers. Cucumbers can be packed in jars with salt, allowing the natural brining process to occur. The cucumbers absorb the salt, creating a flavorful pickle that can be enjoyed year-round. The versatility of pickling vegetables demonstrates the enduring appeal of salt preservation in enhancing flavors and extending the shelf life of seasonal produce.

The cultural significance of salt preservation extends beyond mere survival. Throughout history, salt has held immense value, often being referred to as "white gold." Its ability to preserve food transformed trade and commerce, as salted meats and fish became essential commodities for long-distance travel and trade routes. Salted products were vital for armies, explorers, and merchants, ensuring they had reliable food sources during their journeys.

In addition to its role in trade, salt preservation also fosters community connections. Many cultures have traditional recipes and methods passed down through generations, reflecting a deep-rooted appreciation for food preservation practices. The act of curing meats or pickling vegetables often brings families together, creating a sense of unity and shared heritage.

Today, the practice of salt preservation remains relevant as people seek sustainable methods for storing food. With the resurgence of interest in traditional and artisanal foods, many are turning to salt curing as a way to create unique flavors while honoring time-honored techniques. Home cooks and chefs alike are experimenting with various salt preservation methods, revitalizing the culinary traditions of their ancestors.

Modern innovations in food preservation, such as refrigeration and freezing, have undoubtedly changed the landscape of food storage. However, the principles of salt preservation continue to hold value. Understanding how to use salt effectively allows individuals to embrace self-sufficiency, minimize food waste, and enjoy the rich flavors that come from these ancient practices.

In conclusion, salt preservation is a vital ancient technique for extending the shelf life of meats, fish, and vegetables. Through methods such as dry curing, brining, and pickling, cultures around the world have developed unique recipes and traditions that showcase the art of preservation. By learning and practicing these techniques, we can connect with our culinary heritage while ensuring that our food remains safe, flavorful, and nutritious for the long haul. As we explore the world of salt preservation, we not only honor the wisdom of our ancestors but also cultivate a sustainable approach to food that resonates with modern sensibilities.

Traditional Healing Remedies and Herbal Medicine

Throughout history, herbal medicine has served as a cornerstone of traditional healing practices in cultures worldwide. The use of herbs to prevent illness and promote well-being is rooted in ancient wisdom and continues to inform contemporary approaches to health. Many common herbs, revered for their medicinal properties, have been used for generations to support the body's natural defenses and mitigate the risk of various ailments. Understanding these herbs and their benefits can empower individuals to take charge of their health and integrate natural remedies into their daily lives.

Herbs have been used for their healing properties long before the advent of modern medicine. Ancient civilizations, such as the Egyptians, Greeks, Chinese, and Indigenous peoples, recognized the value of plants in maintaining health. They developed extensive knowledge of local flora and their therapeutic uses, often relying on this wisdom to treat ailments and enhance well-being. This knowledge was passed down through generations, laying the foundation for today's herbal practices.

One of the most widely recognized herbs for illness prevention is **garlic (Allium sativum)**. Garlic has a long history of use as a natural remedy for various ailments. It is known for its potent antibacterial, antiviral, and antifungal properties, making it a powerful ally in boosting the immune system. Allicin, the active compound in garlic, has been shown to enhance the body's immune response and reduce the severity and duration of colds and infections. Incorporating garlic into the diet can help ward off illness, as it can be used in a variety of culinary dishes, from soups to stir-fries, or consumed raw for maximum potency.

Echinacea is another prominent herb renowned for its immune-boosting properties. Native American tribes have used echinacea for centuries to prevent and treat infections, particularly respiratory conditions. The herb is believed to stimulate the production of white blood cells, which play a crucial role in the immune response. Studies suggest that echinacea may reduce the risk of developing colds and flu and can even shorten their duration when taken at the onset of symptoms. Echinacea can be consumed as a tea, tincture, or in capsule form, making it a versatile option for supporting health.

Ginger (Zingiber officinale) is not only a popular culinary spice but also a powerful medicinal herb. It possesses anti-inflammatory and antioxidant properties, making it effective in preventing various illnesses. Ginger is particularly beneficial for digestive health, helping to alleviate nausea and promote overall gastrointestinal function. Its ability to support circulation and enhance immune function makes it a valuable addition to a preventative health regimen. Fresh ginger can be used in teas, smoothies, or as a spice in cooking, while dried ginger powder can be added to baked goods or soups.

Turmeric (Curcuma longa), often referred to as "the golden spice," is well known for its anti-inflammatory properties, largely attributed to its active compound, curcumin. Turmeric has been used in traditional medicine systems, particularly in Ayurveda, for centuries to prevent a variety of health issues. Its potent antioxidant properties help protect the body from oxidative stress and inflammation, contributing to overall well-being. Incorporating turmeric into the diet can be done through curries, golden milk, or as a supplement. Additionally, combining turmeric with black pepper enhances the absorption of curcumin, amplifying its health benefits.

Peppermint (Mentha piperita) is a fragrant herb that has been utilized for its medicinal properties since ancient times. Known for its soothing effects on the digestive system, peppermint can help alleviate symptoms of indigestion, bloating, and nausea. Its antispasmodic properties can also aid in preventing digestive discomfort. Beyond digestive health, peppermint's menthol content has a cooling effect, making it beneficial for headaches and respiratory issues. Drinking peppermint tea or inhaling peppermint oil can provide immediate relief and contribute to overall health.

Chamomile (Matricaria chamomilla) is another common herb celebrated for its calming effects and potential health benefits. Often consumed as a tea, chamomile is known for its ability to promote relaxation, improve sleep quality, and reduce anxiety. Its anti-inflammatory properties may help alleviate symptoms associated with colds and respiratory infections. Regular consumption of chamomile tea can not only serve as a soothing bedtime ritual but also enhance immune function and overall well-being.

Thyme (Thymus vulgaris) is a culinary herb that also offers impressive health benefits. Rich in antioxidants, thyme has antimicrobial properties that can help combat infections and support respiratory health. Thyme oil is often used in herbal remedies for coughs and respiratory conditions, as it helps relax the muscles in the respiratory tract and may aid in clearing mucus. Incorporating thyme into meals or steeping it in hot water for tea can provide a flavorful way to support immune function.

Nettle (Urtica dioica), often regarded as a weed, is a highly nutritious herb with a rich history in traditional medicine. Nettle leaves are packed with vitamins, minerals, and antioxidants, making them beneficial for overall health. Nettle is known to support the immune system and has anti-inflammatory properties. It can be consumed as a tea or added to soups and stews, providing a nutrient boost while helping to prevent illness.

Rosemary (Rosmarinus officinalis) is a fragrant herb commonly used in cooking, but it also offers several health benefits. Rich in antioxidants and anti-inflammatory compounds, rosemary is believed to support cognitive function and protect against oxidative stress. Its antimicrobial properties make it effective in preventing infections and promoting overall health. Rosemary can be used fresh or dried in a variety of dishes, or brewed as a tea for added health benefits.

Holy Basil (Ocimum sanctum), also known as Tulsi, is revered in Ayurvedic medicine for its adaptogenic properties. This herb helps the body adapt to stress and promotes overall balance and well-being. Holy basil is known to enhance immune function, protect against respiratory infections, and reduce inflammation. It can be consumed as a tea or used in cooking, providing both flavor and health benefits.

While the potential benefits of these common herbs for illness prevention are impressive, it is essential to approach their use with mindfulness. Individuals should be aware of any allergies, interactions with medications, or pre-existing health conditions that may affect their ability to use certain herbs safely. Consulting with a healthcare professional or a qualified herbalist can provide guidance on the best practices for incorporating herbs into a wellness routine.

Incorporating these common herbs into one's diet can be a proactive step toward maintaining health and preventing illness. The versatility of these herbs allows for creative culinary applications, from teas and infusions to seasoning dishes. By embracing the wisdom of traditional healing remedies and herbal medicine, individuals can enhance their well-being, connect with nature, and foster a greater understanding of the natural world around them.

In conclusion, common herbs for illness prevention play a vital role in traditional healing practices and contemporary health approaches. The ancient knowledge of herbs such as garlic, echinacea, ginger, turmeric, peppermint, chamomile, thyme, nettle, rosemary, and holy basil underscores the enduring significance of these plants in supporting health and preventing illness. By integrating these herbs into daily life, individuals can take proactive steps toward enhancing their well-being while honoring the rich legacy of herbal medicine that has been passed down through generations. The journey into herbal healing invites exploration, curiosity, and a deeper connection to the natural world, fostering a holistic approach to health that resonates with the wisdom of our ancestors.

The art of preparing herbal remedies such as salves, poultices, and teas has been an integral aspect of traditional healing practices across cultures for centuries. These simple yet effective preparations allow individuals to harness the natural properties of herbs, offering relief from various ailments while promoting overall health and well-being. Understanding how to prepare these remedies not only empowers individuals to take charge of their health but also reconnects them with ancient wisdom that has stood the test of time.

Salves

Salves are thick ointments made from herbs infused in oils, often combined with beeswax to create a soothing topical remedy. They are typically used to alleviate skin conditions, promote wound healing, and provide relief from muscle aches and joint pain. The process of making a salve involves several key steps: selecting the appropriate herbs, infusing them into oil, and combining them with beeswax.

Selecting the Herbs: When choosing herbs for salves, consider their healing properties. Common choices include **calendula** for its anti-inflammatory and healing effects, **chamomile** for its soothing properties, and **arnica** for bruises and muscle pain. Each herb brings unique benefits, so select those that best address the intended purpose of the salve.

Infusing the Oil: The first step in making a salve is to create an herbal oil infusion. This can be done using either the cold infusion method or the heat infusion method. For a cold infusion, place the dried herbs in a jar and cover them with a carrier oil such as olive oil or sweet almond oil. Seal the jar and let it sit in a warm, dark place for about 4 to 6 weeks, shaking it occasionally. The oil will gradually take on the color and fragrance of the herbs.

For a quicker option, use the heat infusion method. Combine the herbs and oil in a double boiler, heating gently for 1 to 3 hours. Ensure the oil does not exceed 120°F (49°C) to preserve the medicinal properties of the herbs. After infusion, strain the oil through a fine mesh strainer or cheesecloth to remove the plant material, leaving you with a fragrant herbal oil.

Combining with Beeswax: To transform the infused oil into a salve, melt beeswax in a double boiler and mix it with the herbal oil. The typical ratio is about 1 part beeswax to 4 parts infused oil, but this can be adjusted based on the desired consistency. Stir the mixture until the beeswax is fully melted and incorporated, then pour it into clean, sterilized containers for storage. Allow the salve to cool and solidify before use. This herbal salve can be applied to minor cuts, scrapes, dry skin, and muscle pain, providing relief and promoting healing.

Poultices

Poultices are another traditional form of herbal remedy, consisting of fresh or dried herbs that are mashed or ground into a paste and applied directly to the skin. They are often used to draw out infections, reduce inflammation, and soothe irritated tissues. Preparing a poultice is a straightforward process that requires minimal ingredients.

Selecting the Herbs: The choice of herbs for a poultice depends on the condition being treated. For example, **plantain** leaves are excellent for drawing out infections, while **comfrey** is known for its healing properties for wounds and bruises. **Mustard** and **ginger** can also be used for their warming properties, making them effective for sore muscles and joint pain.

Preparing the Poultice: To prepare a poultice, begin by crushing fresh herbs using a mortar and pestle or a food processor. If using dried herbs, you can rehydrate them by soaking them in hot water for a few minutes before mashing them into a paste. The consistency should be thick enough to hold together without being too watery.

Once the paste is prepared, spread it onto a clean cloth or gauze, creating a layer about ¼ inch thick. Apply the poultice directly to the affected area of the skin and secure it in place with a bandage or additional cloth. For maximum effectiveness, cover the poultice with plastic wrap to maintain moisture and warmth. Leave it on for about 30 minutes to 2 hours, depending on the severity of the condition being treated.

Teas

Herbal teas are one of the simplest and most popular ways to consume medicinal herbs. Drinking herbal teas can promote hydration, support digestion, and provide various health benefits depending on the chosen ingredients. The preparation of herbal teas typically involves steeping dried or fresh herbs in hot water to extract their flavors and beneficial compounds.

Selecting the Herbs: The selection of herbs for tea will vary based on the desired effects. For calming and relaxation, herbs like **chamomile**, **lavender**, and **lemon balm** are excellent choices. For digestive support, consider **peppermint**, **ginger**, or **fennel**. If seeking immune support, herbs like **echinacea**, **thyme**, and **elderberry** can be included.

Preparing the Tea: To prepare herbal tea, start by boiling water in a kettle or saucepan. While the water is heating, measure out the desired amount of dried or fresh herbs. A general guideline is to use about 1 teaspoon of dried herbs or 1 tablespoon of fresh herbs per cup of water. Place the herbs in a teapot or a heat-safe container.

Once the water reaches a boil, pour it over the herbs and cover the container to trap the steam and essential oils. Allow the tea to steep for about 5 to 15 minutes, depending on the strength desired and the type of herbs used. Longer steeping times can extract more flavors and benefits but may also lead to bitterness in some herbs.

After steeping, strain the tea into a cup, discarding the herbal material. Enjoy the tea warm, and consider adding honey, lemon, or other natural sweeteners to enhance the flavor. Drinking herbal teas regularly can serve as a preventive measure to support overall health and well-being.

The preparation of salves, poultices, and teas embodies the rich tradition of herbal medicine, providing accessible and effective remedies for a variety of ailments. By understanding the properties of different herbs and learning how to prepare these simple yet powerful remedies, individuals can harness the healing potential of nature. These practices not only promote physical health but also encourage a deeper connection with the natural world, fostering a sense of empowerment and self-sufficiency.

Incorporating these herbal preparations into daily life is a way to honor the wisdom of ancient traditions while addressing modern health concerns. As individuals explore the art of herbal medicine, they embark on a journey of discovery, learning to appreciate the healing potential of the plants that surround them. Whether through creating soothing salves, effective poultices, or delightful herbal teas, the benefits of these preparations extend far beyond their immediate applications, enriching the lives of those who embrace the age-old practices of natural healing.

Ancient Practices for Treating Wounds and Infections

Throughout history, the treatment of wounds and infections has been an essential aspect of healthcare. Long before the development of modern medicine and antibiotics, ancient civilizations relied on a combination of knowledge, intuition, and the natural world to heal injuries and combat infections. These practices reflect the resilience and ingenuity of early healers, who drew upon their observations of nature and the medicinal properties of plants. The methods they developed not only highlight their understanding of the human body but also continue to influence contemporary healing approaches. By exploring ancient methods of treating wounds and infections, we can appreciate the profound wisdom embedded in these time-honored traditions and recognize their relevance today.

The historical context of wound care reveals that ancient societies, from the Egyptians and Greeks to Indigenous peoples of North America, recognized the importance of treating injuries effectively. Their observations led to a rich tapestry of healing practices that combined the use of herbs, minerals, and animal products. Ancient Egyptians documented their healing knowledge on papyrus scrolls, detailing the use of honey, oils, and various plant extracts for treating wounds. In many Indigenous cultures, healers, often referred to as shamans or medicine men, played a pivotal role in maintaining community health, utilizing local flora to address injuries and infections.

Herbal remedies were central to ancient wound care. Many plants possess natural antiseptic, anti-inflammatory, and healing properties that have made them invaluable for treating wounds. Honey, for example, is one of the oldest wound treatments known to humanity. Its natural antibacterial properties have been celebrated since ancient times. The Egyptians used honey extensively to treat wounds and prevent infections, leveraging its high sugar content to create a hypertonic environment that inhibits bacterial growth. Additionally, honey's composition includes antioxidants and nutrients that support tissue regeneration. Applying a thin layer of honey to a clean wound can facilitate healing while reducing the risk of infection.

Aloe vera, another plant revered in ancient healing practices, has been used for centuries to soothe and heal wounds. The gel extracted from its leaves is known for its anti-inflammatory and antimicrobial properties, promoting healing by keeping the wound moist and reducing inflammation. Ancient Egyptians referred to aloe as the "plant of immortality," utilizing it to treat various skin ailments, including burns, cuts, and abrasions. To apply aloe vera for wound care, the fresh gel can be extracted from the leaves and gently applied to the affected area, providing both relief and healing support.

Comfrey, often called "knitbone," boasts a long history of use in wound healing. This herb contains allantoin, a compound that promotes cell proliferation and tissue regeneration. Ancient healers used comfrey poultices for a variety of injuries, including fractures, sprains, and wounds. The leaves can be crushed and applied directly to the affected area, or a poultice can be made by mixing dried comfrey with water to create a paste. This preparation not only facilitates healing but also reduces inflammation and pain, making it a valuable remedy for various injuries.

Yarrow has been used for centuries as a wound healer due to its antiseptic properties. The plant contains compounds that promote clotting and reduce inflammation, making it effective in treating cuts and abrasions. Ancient Greeks and Native Americans alike relied on yarrow leaves to staunch bleeding and prevent infection. To use yarrow for wound care, fresh leaves can be crushed and applied directly to the wound, or a tea can be brewed and used as a wash to cleanse the area. This gentle yet effective herb highlights the ancient understanding of the healing properties of plants.

Plantain is a common herb found in gardens and along roadsides, known for its traditional use as a remedy for wounds. With its anti-inflammatory and antimicrobial properties, plantain is effective in treating cuts, insect bites, and stings. The leaves can be chewed to release their juices and then applied directly to the wound, or a poultice can be made by mashing the leaves with a little water. This preparation not only soothes irritation but also reduces swelling and promotes healing.

In addition to herbal remedies, ancient cultures employed various techniques to treat infections and prevent their spread. The importance of cleanliness in wound care was recognized, and healers often used water, vinegar, or herbal infusions to cleanse injuries and remove debris. In some cases, hot water or steam was utilized to disinfect wounds, as heat can kill bacteria and promote blood flow to the area. The practice of debridement, or the removal of dead tissue, was also common, ensuring that wounds could heal properly and reducing the risk of infection.

Natural antiseptics were employed alongside herbal remedies in ancient wound care. For instance, myrrh and frankincense were combined in ancient Egypt and used to create antiseptic mixtures for treating wounds. The use of vinegar as disinfectants was common in many cultures, providing a way to reduce bacterial load on wounds and support the healing process. The understanding of how to create antiseptic solutions from natural sources showcases the depth of ancient healing knowledge.

Ancient healers also understood the importance of protecting wounds from external contaminants. They often used animal skins, cloth, or plant leaves to cover injuries, with the choice of materials dependent on availability and cultural practices. Proper bandaging techniques not only kept the wound clean but also provided support and reduced movement, allowing for optimal healing. Some cultures even developed methods for creating compresses infused with herbs or other healing substances, offering both protection and therapeutic benefits.

Dietary considerations played a significant role in ancient healing practices. Nutrient-rich foods were emphasized to promote recovery and bolster the immune system. Many ancient societies recognized the importance of protein, vitamins, and minerals in the healing process. For example, ancient Romans consumed a diet rich in legumes, fish, and herbs, believing that proper nutrition could aid in recovery from wounds and infections. The holistic understanding of health demonstrated by these cultures underscores the interconnectedness of body, mind, and spirit in the healing process.

Spiritual beliefs and rituals often accompanied ancient practices for treating wounds and infections. Many societies viewed healing as a holistic process that involved not only the physical body but also the emotional and spiritual well-being of the individual. Rituals and ceremonies were commonly performed to invoke healing energies, connect with the divine, or seek the assistance of spirits. This intertwining of spirituality and healing reflects a profound understanding of the human experience, acknowledging that emotional support and spiritual connection can significantly impact physical recovery.

In some Indigenous cultures, shamans or spiritual leaders conducted healing ceremonies that incorporated herbal remedies and spiritual guidance. These rituals often involved music, prayer, and community support, fostering a sense of connection and belonging for the individual receiving care. The social aspect of healing emphasized the importance of compassion, nurturing, and communal support in recovery, illustrating how ancient practices integrated emotional and social dimensions into physical healing.

The ancient methods for treating wounds and infections offer valuable insights that remain relevant today. The resurgence of interest in herbal remedies and natural healing reflects a growing recognition of the efficacy of time-honored traditions. Many contemporary herbalists and natural health practitioners draw upon ancient wisdom, combining it with modern scientific knowledge to create effective treatment protocols for various ailments. The principles of cleanliness, the use of natural antiseptics, and the emphasis on holistic healing are now integral components of many alternative and integrative medicine practices.

While modern medicine has made significant advancements, incorporating natural remedies and practices into healthcare can enhance treatment outcomes and promote overall well-being. The ancient understanding of the healing properties of plants and the significance of community support in recovery provides a holistic approach to health that resonates with contemporary desires for more natural and balanced lifestyles.

In conclusion, the ancient practices for treating wounds and infections reveal a rich tapestry of knowledge cultivated over centuries. The use of herbal remedies, natural antiseptics, and holistic approaches underscores the resilience and resourcefulness of ancient cultures. By understanding and appreciating these practices, individuals can draw upon the wisdom of the past to inform their own health choices, fostering a deeper connection to nature and the healing properties it offers. The exploration of these time-honored practices serves not only as a means of honoring the legacy of traditional healing but also as a way to empower individuals to take an active role in their health and well-being. As we navigate the complexities of modern healthcare, embracing the insights of ancient wisdom can provide a holistic approach to healing that acknowledges our physical, emotional, and spiritual needs. Through this journey, we can cultivate a greater appreciation for the natural world and the profound ways it supports our path to health and wellness.

Water Sourcing and Purification

Water is essential for survival, and throughout history, the ability to find and purify water has been a crucial skill for human beings. Ancient civilizations developed a deep understanding of their environments, enabling them to locate safe water sources and implement methods for purification. The significance of water in ancient societies cannot be overstated; it was fundamental not only for hydration but also for agriculture, sanitation, and overall community health. This exploration of how ancient peoples identified and accessed safe water sources reveals not only their resourcefulness but also their profound connection to the natural world.

The quest for safe drinking water begins with the ability to recognize potential water sources in the environment. Ancient cultures learned to observe the landscape and identify signs that indicated the presence of water. Rivers, streams, lakes, and springs were primary sources of water. Early humans were adept at reading the land; they recognized that valleys often harbored streams and that certain types of vegetation, such as willows and rushes, tended to grow near water. Such observations were crucial for locating water, especially in arid regions where surface water might be scarce.

In addition to natural sources, ancient peoples understood the importance of seasonal changes in their environment. Many relied on their knowledge of weather patterns and seasonal rains to locate temporary water sources, such as puddles or pools that formed after rainfall. They would scout their surroundings during periods of rainfall to identify areas that could hold water for later use. This seasonal awareness was vital for survival, as it enabled communities to gather and store water before it dried up.

Another method employed by ancient peoples to locate water was the study of animal behavior. Animals instinctively seek out water sources, and observing their movements often provided valuable clues for humans. For instance, certain birds, like herons and ducks, are indicators of nearby water. Animals also tend to create paths to their watering holes, making their trails useful for finding hidden sources of water. Ancient hunters and gatherers would follow these trails, knowing that they would lead them to life-sustaining resources.

In addition to identifying surface water, ancient cultures often found innovative ways to access groundwater. Digging wells was a common practice in many ancient societies. By carefully excavating into the ground, they could reach the water table and tap into a reliable source of water. Well construction techniques varied across regions, depending on local geology and the availability of materials. In some areas, ancient peoples lined their wells with stones to prevent collapse, while in others, they used clay to seal the walls and minimize contamination.

Spring water, which emerges from underground aquifers, was highly prized for its purity. Many ancient cultures revered springs as sacred sites, believing they were sources of life and healing. Springs often bubbled up through natural rock formations, creating pools of clear water. The ancient Greeks, for example, established rituals and shrines around springs, highlighting their significance in both daily life and spiritual practices. To access spring water, people would typically travel to these natural sites, recognizing that the water was naturally filtered and less likely to be contaminated than water from stagnant sources.

Once water sources were identified and accessed, purification methods became crucial for ensuring its safety for consumption. Ancient peoples relied on a variety of techniques to purify water, many of which are still relevant today. One of the simplest methods involved the use of natural filtration. In areas with sandy or gravelly soil, individuals would create makeshift filters by digging a small pit and layering it with different materials, such as stones, charcoal, and sand. Water would then be poured through these layers, allowing impurities and sediments to be trapped, resulting in cleaner water. This method, while rudimentary, demonstrated an early understanding of filtration principles.

Boiling water was another effective purification technique employed by ancient cultures. The process of boiling not only kills harmful pathogens but also helps remove impurities. Ancient peoples recognized the value of heat in water purification and often built fires to bring water to a rolling boil. This technique was especially useful when accessing surface water from ponds or rivers, where contamination from animal waste or decaying organic matter could pose significant health risks. Boiling water until it reached a safe temperature was a practical method that ensured its safety for drinking and cooking.

In addition to boiling and filtration, various natural substances were used to further purify water. For instance, certain plants, such as the leaves of the moringa tree, have been shown to possess coagulating properties, making them effective in clarifying water. The seeds of the moringa tree can be crushed and added to water, where they attract and bind impurities, allowing them to settle at the bottom. This ancient practice of using plant materials for water purification reflects the deep knowledge that early peoples had regarding the natural properties of their environment.

Ancient civilizations also employed methods for storing water to ensure its availability during dry seasons or emergencies. Cisterns and clay pots were commonly used to collect and store rainwater. These storage methods helped conserve water for later use and were often built in areas where surface water was scarce. Communities developed intricate systems for collecting rainwater from roofs and directing it into storage vessels. This practice not only demonstrated their resourcefulness but also highlighted their understanding of the importance of water conservation.

The cultural significance of water sourcing and purification cannot be overlooked. Many ancient societies incorporated water into their spiritual practices and rituals, emphasizing its life-giving qualities. Sacred wells, springs, and rivers were often associated with deities or spirits, and the act of drawing water was imbued with reverence and respect. Communities would come together to celebrate rituals surrounding water, recognizing its role in sustaining life and fostering a sense of unity.

As we reflect on the ancient practices of identifying and accessing safe water sources, we gain insight into the profound wisdom embedded in these traditions. The ability to locate and purify water was not merely a survival skill; it was a vital component of community health and well-being. By observing the land, understanding animal behavior, and utilizing natural resources, ancient peoples demonstrated remarkable adaptability and resilience in the face of environmental challenges.

In contemporary society, where modern technology provides easy access to clean water, it is essential to remember the lessons learned from our ancestors. The ancient practices of water sourcing and purification remind us of the importance of water conservation and the need to respect and protect our water sources. As we face the challenges of climate change and increasing water scarcity, revisiting these time-honored methods can inspire sustainable practices that honor the interconnectedness of humans and the natural world.

Ultimately, the journey of identifying and accessing safe water sources reflects humanity's enduring quest for survival and connection to nature. By understanding and embracing these ancient practices, we can cultivate a deeper appreciation for water's significance in our lives and foster a sense of stewardship toward this precious resource. As we navigate the complexities of modern living, let us draw inspiration from the wisdom of those who came before us, recognizing that the lessons of the past can guide us toward a more sustainable and harmonious future.

Purification Techniques without Modern Filters

Water is a fundamental necessity for life, and ensuring its purity has been a priority for humans throughout history. Before the advent of modern filtration systems, ancient civilizations developed a variety of ingenious techniques to purify water, relying on natural materials and methods available in their environments. These techniques not only demonstrate the resourcefulness of our ancestors but also reveal a deep understanding of the properties of water and the materials used for purification. In this exploration, we will delve into several traditional methods of water purification that were employed by ancient peoples, showcasing their effectiveness and ingenuity.

One of the simplest and most widely used techniques for purifying water is boiling. This method harnesses the power of heat to kill harmful microorganisms, making water safe for consumption. Ancient peoples recognized that boiling water could effectively eliminate pathogens that could cause illness. The process involves heating water until it reaches a rolling boil and maintaining that temperature for a specific duration—typically a minimum of five to ten minutes. This method was particularly important for purifying water sourced from rivers, lakes, or ponds, where contamination from animals or decaying organic matter could occur.

Boiling not only ensures the microbial safety of water but also enhances its taste. This technique has been passed down through generations and is still a fundamental practice in many cultures around the world. The use of fire pits, hearths, or other primitive cooking methods to boil water demonstrates the practicality of this approach in ancient societies. In times of scarcity, boiling also provided a way to make unpalatable water sources drinkable, allowing communities to survive during challenging conditions.

Another effective purification technique employed by ancient peoples was natural filtration. This method involved using layers of natural materials to filter out impurities from water. Ancient cultures observed that certain materials, such as sand, gravel, charcoal, and plant fibers, had filtering properties that could remove sediments, debris, and even some pathogens from water. To create a natural filter, individuals would dig a shallow pit and layer it with these materials in specific order, starting with larger particles like gravel at the bottom and gradually moving to finer materials like sand and charcoal at the top.

Water would then be poured through this filtration system, allowing it to pass through the layers and emerge cleaner and clearer. The charcoal, in particular, played a crucial role in absorbing impurities and improving taste. This method was not only effective but also easily adaptable, as it could be constructed using readily available resources found in the local environment. By utilizing natural filtration techniques, ancient peoples demonstrated a practical understanding of the physical and chemical properties of materials that enhanced the safety and palatability of their water.

In addition to boiling and filtration, ancient cultures often utilized solar purification methods. This technique harnesses the power of the sun's ultraviolet rays to disinfect water. The process involves filling clear containers, such as glass or clay jars, with contaminated water and placing them in direct sunlight for several hours, ideally on a sunny day. The heat and UV rays work together to kill harmful microorganisms, making the water safer to drink.

Solar purification is especially effective in regions where sunlight is abundant, and it offers a sustainable solution for water purification without the need for fuel or complex systems. This method was widely used in various cultures, particularly in areas with limited access to firewood or other fuel sources. The simplicity of this technique highlights the resourcefulness of ancient peoples, who often adapted their methods to suit the environmental conditions they faced.

Sedimentation is another ancient purification method that relies on the natural settling of particles in water. This technique involves allowing water to sit undisturbed for a period of time, during which heavier particles and sediments settle to the bottom of the container. Once the sediment has settled, the clearer water can be carefully poured or siphoned off, leaving the contaminants behind. While sedimentation may not eliminate pathogens, it is an effective way to reduce turbidity and improve the clarity of water.

This method was particularly useful in situations where water was collected from rivers or streams that may have carried silt, mud, or other debris. Ancient peoples often combined sedimentation with other purification techniques, such as boiling or filtration, to enhance the overall safety of the water. By understanding the natural properties of water and utilizing simple physical processes, ancient cultures effectively improved the quality of their drinking water.

Activated charcoal has been utilized for centuries as a powerful natural purifier. While it was likely discovered by ancient peoples through trial and error, the effectiveness of charcoal in removing impurities from water has been well-documented. To create activated charcoal, hardwood is burned at high temperatures in a low-oxygen environment, resulting in a porous material with a large surface area. This porous structure allows charcoal to adsorb a wide range of contaminants, including bacteria, chemicals, and unpleasant tastes or odors.

Ancient societies often used charcoal in combination with other filtration methods. For instance, water would be poured through layers of sand and charcoal to enhance purification. The charcoal not only helped improve the taste and clarity of the water but also acted as a natural disinfectant. Ancient Egyptians, for example, used charcoal as a part of their water treatment processes, showcasing its importance in maintaining health and hygiene in their communities.

The practice of using natural coagulants was also prevalent among ancient cultures. Certain plants and minerals possess coagulant properties that can help to clarify water by causing impurities to clump together and settle. One well-known natural coagulant is the seed of the moringa tree, which has been used for centuries in various cultures. The seeds can be crushed into a powder and added to turbid water, where they bind with suspended particles, allowing them to settle at the bottom.

Once the impurities have settled, the clearer water can be decanted, leaving behind the contaminants. This technique not only demonstrates an understanding of water purification but also reflects the deep knowledge that ancient peoples had regarding their local flora and fauna. The use of natural coagulants exemplifies the integration of science and tradition in ancient water purification practices.

While these ancient purification techniques may seem rudimentary by today's standards, they underscore the importance of water safety and the innovative spirit of humanity. The methods employed by our ancestors highlight their resilience and adaptability in the face of environmental challenges. In many ways, these ancient techniques are not only relevant but also essential in contemporary discussions about water sustainability, particularly in regions facing water scarcity or contamination.

In modern times, as we grapple with the challenges of water pollution and scarcity, revisiting these ancient purification techniques can inspire sustainable practices that honor the interconnectedness of humans and the environment. By learning from our ancestors, we can cultivate a deeper appreciation for the resources available to us and promote responsible water management.

Ultimately, the ancient methods of water purification serve as a reminder that even in the absence of modern technology, human ingenuity and a profound understanding of nature can lead to effective solutions for survival. As we explore and implement these techniques today, we not only pay homage to our ancestors but also ensure the continued health and well-being of our communities and the planet.

Building Basic Water Storage Systems

Water storage is a crucial aspect of survival, particularly in environments where water scarcity is a concern. Throughout history, ancient civilizations have developed various methods and systems to effectively store water for both daily use and emergency situations. These systems not only ensured a reliable water supply but also showcased the ingenuity of our ancestors in utilizing available materials and resources. In this discussion, we will explore the fundamentals of building basic water storage systems, examining traditional techniques and structures that have stood the test of time.

One of the simplest and most effective methods for water storage is the use of containers made from natural materials. In ancient times, people utilized clay, wood, and stone to create water-holding vessels. Clay pots, in particular, have been used for thousands of years due to their availability and ability to keep water cool. The porous nature of unglazed clay allows for a degree of evaporation, which can help lower the temperature of the water inside, making it more palatable.

To construct a basic clay pot, artisans would gather local clay and shape it into a vessel using techniques such as coiling or molding. Once shaped, the pots would be dried in the sun or fired in a kiln to harden them. Ancient peoples often decorated these pots, which also served practical purposes, such as reinforcing the structure or providing a means of identification for different water sources.

While clay pots are effective for small-scale water storage, larger systems are often required for communities or agricultural purposes. One such system is the construction of cisterns or water reservoirs. These structures are designed to collect and store rainwater, providing a sustainable water source during dry periods. Ancient cultures in arid regions, such as the Romans and the Maya, developed sophisticated cistern systems that utilized gravity to direct water into storage.

To build a basic cistern, the first step involves selecting an appropriate location, ideally one that can capture rainwater runoff. The site should be cleared of debris and any vegetation that could contaminate the water. Next, a trench is excavated to create a basin, which is typically lined with stones or clay to prevent seepage.

Once the basin is ready, a roof or covering is often constructed to minimize evaporation and prevent debris from entering the cistern. This covering can be made from thatch, wooden beams, or stone slabs, depending on the available materials. In some cases, a simple funnel system may be created to direct rainwater into the cistern, enhancing its efficiency.

The design of cisterns varies among cultures, but the underlying principle remains the same: to capture and store water efficiently. In regions where rainfall is sporadic, cisterns provided a vital resource for drinking, irrigation, and livestock. The construction of these systems exemplifies the resourcefulness of ancient peoples and their ability to adapt to their environments.

In addition to cisterns, ancient civilizations also utilized various earthworks to create water storage systems. Earthworks, such as terraces and check dams, are designed to slow down water runoff and promote infiltration into the soil. By building terraces on hillsides, ancient farmers were able to capture and store rainwater, enhancing soil moisture and improving crop yields.

To create terraces, communities would dig shallow channels into the hillside, following the natural contours of the land. These channels would help direct water flow, allowing it to settle and permeate into the soil rather than running off into streams and rivers. This method not only conserved water but also reduced soil erosion, contributing to long-term agricultural sustainability.

Check dams are another type of earthwork designed to capture water and create small reservoirs. These structures are built across small streams or gullies, slowing down water flow and allowing it to pool behind the dam. Over time, this pooling can create small ponds or wetlands, which serve as vital habitats for wildlife and sources of water for nearby communities. The construction of check dams exemplifies the ancient understanding of hydrology and the importance of managing water resources effectively.

Traditional methods of creating water storage systems often included the use of reeds or other aquatic plants. In regions where freshwater sources were abundant, ancient peoples discovered that large containers made from reeds could be used to store water effectively. These containers, known as "reeds boats," were crafted by weaving reeds together to create a buoyant structure that could hold water.

To construct a reed boat for water storage, individuals would gather long, flexible reeds and weave them into a watertight vessel. These boats could be used not only for transporting water but also for storing it temporarily while transporting it from one location to another. The lightweight nature of reed boats allowed for easy movement, making them an ideal solution for communities that relied on waterways for their water supply.

In addition to these methods, the use of animal skins or bladders for water storage has a long history in many cultures. Animal skins, particularly those of goats and sheep, were often treated and sewn together to create water bags that could hold liquids. These bags were portable, making them useful for nomadic societies or during travel.

The construction of animal skin water bags involved careful preparation. The skins would be cleaned and cured to prevent spoilage. Once treated, they would be shaped into bags and sealed at the edges, creating a durable container for holding water. While not as long-lasting as clay or stone vessels, these water bags offered a practical solution for storing water in the short term.

Ancient peoples also recognized the importance of water quality when constructing storage systems. To maintain the cleanliness of stored water, many cultures employed methods to reduce contamination. For example, some communities placed stones or charcoal in their water containers to absorb impurities and improve taste. This understanding of natural materials and their properties contributed to the effectiveness of ancient water storage systems.

As we examine these ancient water storage techniques, it becomes clear that they were not merely practical solutions; they also embodied a profound relationship between humans and their environment. The construction of water storage systems required careful observation, experimentation, and an understanding of local ecology. Ancient peoples adapted their methods to suit their specific needs, utilizing the resources available to them while respecting the delicate balance of nature.

In modern times, the principles of ancient water storage can still be applied to contemporary water management practices. As communities face increasing challenges related to water scarcity and climate change, revisiting these traditional techniques can provide valuable insights for sustainable water management.

In conclusion, building basic water storage systems is an essential skill that has been practiced by humanity for millennia. From simple clay pots to sophisticated cisterns and earthworks, ancient peoples developed a range of techniques to effectively capture, store, and preserve water. These methods reflect not only the resourcefulness and ingenuity of our ancestors but also their deep understanding of the natural world. By learning from these traditional practices, we can promote sustainable water management and ensure access to clean water for future generations.

Ancient Hunting and Fishing Techniques

Crafting Primitive Traps and Snares

Hunting and fishing are integral aspects of survival that have sustained humanity for millennia. While modern hunting methods often rely on sophisticated technology and equipment, ancient cultures developed a remarkable array of primitive traps and snares that exemplified their ingenuity and deep understanding of animal behavior. These techniques were not only effective in capturing food but also reflected the profound relationship between ancient peoples and their environments. In this exploration, we will delve into the various methods of crafting primitive traps and snares, emphasizing the materials, techniques, and strategies employed by our ancestors.

At the heart of primitive trapping lies the ability to understand animal movements and behaviors. Ancient hunters closely observed their prey, noting patterns in their habits, feeding times, and travel routes. This intimate knowledge of the natural world enabled them to create traps that would effectively exploit these patterns, ensuring a higher likelihood of success. The design of traps and snares varied widely among cultures, depending on the local fauna, available materials, and environmental conditions.

One of the simplest yet most effective primitive traps is the pitfall trap. This type of trap is designed to conceal a deep hole in the ground, which unsuspecting animals may fall into as they move through their territory. To construct a pitfall trap, hunters would first select an appropriate location, often along well-worn animal paths or near feeding areas. The pit is then dug to a depth of several feet, and the sides may be reinforced with stones or logs to prevent escape.

To camouflage the pit, hunters would cover it with a layer of branches, leaves, and other natural materials, creating a false surface that appears solid. The key to a successful pitfall trap is ensuring that it is both hidden and placed strategically along an animal's route. When an unsuspecting animal steps onto the concealed surface, it falls into the pit, rendering it trapped and vulnerable.

Snares, another vital component of primitive trapping, are designed to capture animals alive or incapacitated. A snare typically consists of a noose made from flexible materials such as plant fibers, vines, or animal sinew, attached to a tensioned trigger mechanism. This mechanism can be as simple as a bent sapling or a lever system, designed to pull the noose tight when an animal enters the trap.

To craft a basic snare, hunters would begin by selecting a suitable location along a known animal trail. They would then create a loop with their noose, ensuring it is the appropriate size for the target animal. The snare is anchored to the ground or a sturdy branch, and the trigger mechanism is set up nearby. When the animal attempts to pass through the loop, the trigger is activated, pulling the noose tight around its body or neck. This method can effectively capture animals ranging from rabbits to larger game, depending on the size of the snare.

One of the more sophisticated snare designs is the "figure-four" trap, which incorporates a simple lever and a pivoting system to create a rapid, snapping motion. This trap is particularly effective for larger animals and can be constructed using sticks and branches found in the surrounding environment. The figure-four trap consists of three primary components: the base, the upright stick, and the trigger stick.

To construct the trap, hunters would start by creating a base using a flat piece of wood or stone to support the entire structure. Next, a vertical stick is placed on the base, secured at the bottom with a notched horizontal stick that serves as a pivot point. A trigger stick is then positioned above the vertical stick, holding a heavy weight or a horizontal stick that will fall when the trap is triggered.

When an animal disturbs the trigger stick, the weight falls, causing the upright stick to pivot rapidly downward and strike the animal. This trap requires careful placement and calibration to ensure the right balance and sensitivity, but it exemplifies the clever engineering of ancient trapping techniques.

For smaller animals, the "deadfall" trap is a commonly used primitive method. This trap utilizes a heavy weight, such as a rock or log, suspended above the ground, held in place by a trigger mechanism. When an animal disturbs the bait or triggers the mechanism, the weight drops, crushing or incapacitating the animal beneath it.

To construct a deadfall trap, hunters would begin by digging a shallow hole to secure the weight, ensuring it would fall straight down. A sturdy base is created to hold the weight in place, and a trigger stick is carefully positioned so that the animal must pull on bait placed at the end of the stick. When the animal interacts with the bait, the trigger is released, and the weight drops with significant force.

In addition to traps and snares, ancient peoples developed various techniques to enhance their hunting efficiency. Baiting, for example, is a common strategy employed to lure animals into traps. Hunters often used scents or food that appealed to specific species, strategically placing the bait to increase the likelihood of a catch. This technique requires knowledge of the target animal's diet and habits, allowing hunters to optimize their traps for success.

Fishing techniques also intersect with trapping methods, with many ancient cultures employing similar principles to catch fish. One traditional fishing method is the use of fish traps or weirs, which are barriers placed in rivers or streams to funnel fish into a confined area. These structures can be crafted from local materials such as sticks, stones, and reeds, creating a series of obstacles that guide fish into traps or nets.

To build a fish trap, hunters would first assess the flow of the water and identify areas where fish were likely to congregate, such as shallow pools or bends in the river. They would then construct a series of barriers to create a funnel effect, directing the fish towards a designated catching area. These traps could be left unattended for extended periods, allowing for passive fishing while hunters pursued other activities.

Another effective fishing technique is the use of spears or harpoons, which enable hunters to catch fish directly in the water. Ancient peoples crafted these tools from sturdy wood or bone, often with sharpened tips for increased effectiveness. Skilled fishermen would wade into shallow waters or construct platforms to enhance their reach, employing stealth and patience to spear fish as they swam by.

Throughout history, ancient cultures have shared knowledge and techniques related to trapping and fishing, passing down wisdom from generation to generation. This transmission of knowledge was crucial for survival, as it allowed communities to adapt their methods based on local resources and environmental conditions. Many of these practices are still relevant today, serving as valuable lessons in sustainability and self-sufficiency.

In conclusion, crafting primitive traps and snares is a testament to human ingenuity and adaptability in the pursuit of survival. The ability to understand animal behavior, combined with resourcefulness in using available materials, enabled ancient peoples to effectively capture food and sustain their communities. Whether through pitfall traps, snares, or fishing techniques, these methods exemplify the deep connection between humans and the natural world.

As we look to the future, embracing these ancient practices can inspire modern approaches to hunting, fishing, and food sourcing. By learning from our ancestors, we can cultivate a deeper appreciation for the resources available to us and promote sustainable practices that honor the delicate balance of nature. Ultimately, the art of crafting primitive traps and snares reflects a timeless understanding of survival, resilience, and our enduring relationship with the Earth.

Fishing has been a vital source of sustenance for humanity throughout history, providing not only nourishment but also a connection to the natural world. Among the various methods of fishing, spearfishing and handline fishing stand out as ancient techniques that reflect the ingenuity and adaptability of our ancestors. These methods require minimal equipment, allowing people to engage directly with their environment and harvest fish in a sustainable manner. This exploration delves into the intricacies of spearfishing and handline fishing techniques, examining their historical significance, methods, and the skills required to master them.

Spearfishing, as a technique, dates back thousands of years and is one of the oldest forms of fishing practiced by humans. It involves using a spear or spear-like weapon to catch fish, either in shallow waters or from underwater. The beauty of spearfishing lies in its simplicity and the skill involved, as it demands a keen sense of observation, patience, and precision.

To successfully spearfish, one must first understand the behavior of the target fish species. Knowledge of their feeding habits, preferred habitats, and swimming patterns is essential. Many ancient cultures employed this knowledge, observing fish behavior and seasonal patterns to optimize their chances of a successful catch. Fishermen often waited patiently near reefs, rocks, or underwater structures where fish congregate, relying on their ability to blend into the environment and remain unnoticed.

The construction of spears has evolved over time, with ancient peoples using materials available in their surroundings. Early spears were typically crafted from sturdy wood, often pointed with sharpened stone, bone, or metal tips. The length and design of the spear could vary depending on the target species and fishing conditions. For example, longer spears might be used for larger fish in deeper waters, while shorter spears were more suitable for smaller fish in shallow coastal areas.

A popular technique among spearfishers is the use of a speargun, which employs a mechanical mechanism to propel the spear at high speed. Although this technology is more modern, it builds upon ancient practices and provides greater efficiency in capturing fish. Many spearfishers today still prefer traditional polespears, a long spear without mechanical assistance, as they appreciate the challenge and connection to nature it provides.

When spearfishing, it is common to practice breath-hold diving, a technique that requires the fisherman to descend underwater and remain submerged for a period. This skill involves developing the ability to hold one's breath, manage buoyancy, and navigate underwater environments effectively. Spearfishers often learn to control their movements to minimize disturbances, as sudden motions can frighten fish away. The art of stealth is crucial, as a quiet approach allows the fisherman to get close to their quarry.

In addition to breath-hold diving, some cultures have developed specialized techniques for spearfishing in deeper waters. One such method is known as "free diving," where fishermen descend to significant depths to target larger species. Free divers often utilize weights or belts to assist with sinking and may employ safety lines to prevent losing their way. This method requires extensive training, experience, and awareness of the underwater environment, making it both challenging and rewarding.

Handline fishing is another ancient technique that complements spearfishing and involves using a simple fishing line without the need for a fishing rod or reel. This method allows fishermen to catch fish directly from the surface or in shallow waters, making it accessible to various communities. Handline fishing has a rich history and is still practiced worldwide, particularly in coastal regions where traditional fishing methods persist.

To engage in handline fishing, fishermen typically use a length of strong fishing line attached to a hook, which may be baited with natural lures such as worms, small fish, or squid. The simplicity of handline fishing allows for a direct connection to the water, and fishermen often cast their lines from boats, shorelines, or piers. This method can be effective for catching various species, including snapper, grouper, and other bottom-dwelling fish.

The technique involves a rhythmic process of casting and reeling in the line, allowing fishermen to feel for any bites or tugs. Patience and attentiveness are essential, as the fisherman must remain alert to the movements of the fish below. Many handline fishers develop a keen sense of timing and pressure, learning to distinguish between different fish species based on their biting patterns.

One of the advantages of handline fishing is its adaptability to different environments. Fishermen can modify their techniques based on the available fish species, local conditions, and weather patterns. For instance, during seasonal migrations, handline fishers may change their bait and techniques to target specific fish that are more abundant at certain times of the year.

In addition to traditional handline fishing, many cultures have developed unique variations of the technique. Some fishermen use multiple lines or "handlines" to increase their chances of catching fish. This method involves baiting several hooks on individual lines and casting them simultaneously, creating a spread of lures that can attract fish from different directions.

Both spearfishing and handline fishing embody sustainable practices that align with ancient principles of living in harmony with nature. These methods promote a deep respect for the environment and its resources, encouraging communities to engage in responsible fishing practices. Many ancient cultures believed in the concept of reciprocity with nature, viewing fish not merely as a resource to exploit but as living beings deserving of respect. This philosophy has contributed to the sustainability of these fishing practices over generations.

Moreover, the skills developed through spearfishing and handline fishing extend beyond the act of catching fish. Fishermen cultivate an awareness of their surroundings, learning to read the water, understand weather patterns, and navigate various ecosystems. These skills are invaluable, fostering a connection to the natural world that promotes stewardship and conservation.

As modern society faces increasing challenges related to overfishing and environmental degradation, revisiting these ancient fishing techniques offers valuable insights for sustainable practices. By embracing the principles of spearfishing and handline fishing, contemporary fishers can promote responsible fishing habits, ensuring the health of aquatic ecosystems for future generations.

In conclusion, spearfishing and handline fishing techniques represent the rich heritage of human ingenuity in the pursuit of sustenance. These ancient practices reflect a deep understanding of fish behavior, ecological balance, and the materials available in the environment. As we learn from our ancestors and integrate their wisdom into modern practices, we can cultivate a greater appreciation for our connection to nature and the importance of sustainable fishing methods. The art of fishing, whether through the precision of spearfishing or the simplicity of handline techniques, continues to inspire and teach us about our place within the intricate web of life.

Processing and Cooking Wild Game

The hunting of wild game is a time-honored tradition that connects humanity to its primal roots, fostering a deep appreciation for nature and the life it sustains. The skills involved in processing and cooking wild game are as essential as the hunt itself, encompassing a wealth of knowledge passed down through generations. This topic delves into the art and science of processing wild game, exploring the techniques, tools, and culinary practices that transform fresh meat into nourishing meals. From field dressing immediately after a successful hunt to preparing various cuts for cooking, this process requires careful attention to detail, respect for the animal, and an understanding of the best cooking methods to maximize flavor and tenderness.

Processing wild game begins the moment the animal is harvested. Field dressing is the first crucial step, which involves removing the internal organs to preserve the meat's quality and prevent spoilage. This process requires a steady hand, a sharp knife, and a clear understanding of anatomy to avoid puncturing the intestines or bladder, which could taint the meat. Traditionally, hunters would use a knife made from stone, bone, or metal, often crafted specifically for the task at hand.

Once the game is down, the hunter must find a suitable location to begin field dressing. Ideally, this should be a clean, open area away from potential contaminants. The hunter starts by hanging the animal from its hind legs or placing it on a clean surface. A common technique for field dressing is the "ventral cut," where a small incision is made at the base of the ribcage and extended down to the pelvis. This cut allows the hunter to access the abdominal cavity. Care must be taken to cut just deep enough to avoid damaging organs while ensuring easy access to remove them.

After the initial cut, the next step involves carefully cutting through the connective tissues and ligaments that hold the internal organs in place. The organs can be removed in one motion, or individually, depending on the size of the animal and the hunter's preference. For larger game like deer or elk, it may be more efficient to remove the organs together. During this process, it's essential to keep the meat clean and free of contaminants. Hunters often use a cloth or bandana to wipe away blood and debris.

Once field dressing is complete, the next phase involves skinning the animal. This step not only prepares the meat for cooking but also maximizes the utility of the harvested animal by allowing the hide to be preserved for other uses. Skinning can be done using a sharp knife, taking care to make clean cuts along the legs and neck to avoid tearing the hide. The skin is then peeled away from the flesh, and the knife is used to separate it from the meat at the joints.

Depending on the skill level of the hunter, skinning may take some practice, but it is an essential skill to master for anyone involved in hunting.

After skinning, the meat must be cooled as quickly as possible to prevent spoilage. This often involves hanging the carcass in a cool, shaded area or placing it in a cooler with ice. Aging the meat can enhance its flavor and tenderness, allowing enzymes to break down muscle fibers. The ideal aging period depends on the species and environmental conditions, but many hunters recommend aging deer for a few days to a week, depending on temperature. During this time, the hunter can prepare the meat for cooking or storage.

When it comes to cooking wild game, the techniques and methods can vary widely based on the type of animal and the desired outcome. Wild game is often leaner than domesticated meat, which can lead to a different cooking approach. One of the most effective methods for cooking wild game is slow cooking or braising, which allows the meat to become tender while infusing flavors from herbs, spices, and liquids. This method is particularly suitable for tougher cuts, such as shoulder or leg meat, which benefit from prolonged cooking times.

Marinating wild game before cooking can also help to enhance tenderness and flavor. A marinade can be made from a combination of acidic ingredients, such as vinegar or citrus juice, along with oil, herbs, and spices. The acid helps to break down the muscle fibers, making the meat more tender. Depending on the type of game, different marinades may be suitable. For instance, a marinade with garlic, rosemary works well for venison, while a citrus-based marinade can complement the flavors of wild fowl.

Grilling is another popular method for cooking wild game, especially for tender cuts like steaks or loins. Grilling over an open flame not only imparts a distinct smoky flavor but also seals in the juices, creating a succulent dish. It's important to keep an eye on the cooking time, as wild game can easily overcook due to its lower fat content. Using a meat thermometer can help ensure that the meat is cooked to the desired level of doneness without drying it out.

For those who prefer a more traditional approach, roasting is an excellent option for larger cuts of meat. Roasting involves cooking the meat in an oven at a relatively high temperature, which helps to develop a crispy exterior while keeping the interior juicy. Basting the meat with its own juices or a marinade during the cooking process can add extra flavor and moisture. Cooking times will vary depending on the size and type of the animal, so it's essential to follow recommended cooking times for different species.

Stews and soups are also ideal for utilizing wild game, especially when using tougher cuts or leftover pieces. The slow cooking process allows the flavors to meld together while tenderizing the meat. A classic wild game stew can be prepared by browning chunks of meat in a pot, adding vegetables, herbs, and broth, and simmering until everything is tender. This method not only provides a hearty meal but also reduces waste by making use of all parts of the animal.

When it comes to serving wild game, presentation can enhance the dining experience. Simple garnishes like fresh herbs or a drizzle of sauce can elevate the dish, while traditional side dishes, such as roasted vegetables or wild rice, can complement the flavors of the meat. Pairing wild game with seasonal ingredients can create a well-rounded meal that pays homage to the natural world.

Additionally, cooking wild game encourages a deeper appreciation for the ethical considerations of hunting. The process of harvesting an animal for food connects individuals to the land and the cycles of nature, fostering a sense of responsibility for the environment. Sharing meals made from wild game often strengthens community ties, as families and friends come together to celebrate the fruits of their labor.

In conclusion, processing and cooking wild game encompasses a range of skills and techniques that reflect the enduring relationship between humans and nature. From field dressing to cooking methods, each step is an opportunity to honor the animal and the environment it comes from. As we embrace these ancient practices, we not only enrich our culinary experiences but also cultivate a deeper respect for the resources that sustain us. Whether enjoyed in solitude or shared with loved ones, meals made from wild game serve as a reminder of the connection between hunter, food, and the natural world.

Primitive Cooking and Nutrition

Cooking with fire and hot stones represents one of humanity's earliest culinary techniques, transcending cultures and time periods. This ancient practice not only provided a means to prepare food but also transformed the way early humans interacted with their environment. By harnessing fire and utilizing natural materials, our ancestors developed cooking methods that enhanced flavors, improved digestibility, and offered a safer way to consume a variety of foods. The exploration of cooking with fire and hot stones reveals the ingenuity of early peoples and underscores the vital role these techniques played in their survival and nutrition.

The use of fire for cooking is a fundamental aspect of human evolution. While the precise moment when our ancestors first tamed fire is still a subject of study, it is widely believed to have occurred over a million years ago. Early humans likely discovered the benefits of cooking by observing natural wildfires or scavenging remains from animals that had been inadvertently charred. This pivotal moment allowed for a dramatic shift in diet and lifestyle, as cooked food became more accessible, nutritious, and palatable.

Cooking with fire fundamentally alters the chemical structure of food, making it easier to digest and enhancing nutrient absorption. For instance, the process of cooking breaks down complex carbohydrates and proteins, reducing the time and energy required for digestion. This ability to extract more nutrients from food sources may have played a crucial role in the development of the human brain and overall health. Moreover, the heat of the fire kills harmful bacteria and parasites, making food safer to consume, and thus contributing to improved health outcomes in early human populations.

One of the most straightforward methods of cooking with fire involves open flames. This technique is widely recognized and employed across various cultures. To begin, early cooks would gather dry wood and kindling to create a fire, often in a designated pit or a stone circle. Once a steady flame was established, different cooking methods could be employed, including roasting, baking, and boiling.

Roasting is perhaps the simplest and most ancient form of cooking with fire. Early humans would skewer meat on sticks or place whole animals near the flames, allowing the heat to penetrate the flesh and impart a smoky flavor. This technique not only cooked the meat but also rendered fat, making it an energy-dense food source. The flavors created by roasting over an open fire are often considered some of the most appealing and are still widely celebrated in modern culinary practices.

Another essential method of cooking with fire is baking. While traditional ovens were not available in ancient times, early peoples often used hot stones or heated clay vessels to bake food. By placing dough or other ingredients on flat stones that had been heated in the fire, they could create flatbreads or other baked goods. The use of stones not only provided even heat but also added a unique texture and flavor to the final product.

Boiling, on the other hand, presents a more complex challenge but was nonetheless practiced by early humans. To boil food, they would heat water in containers made from materials like clay or animal hides. Once the water reached the desired temperature, food such as vegetables or grains could be added. However, since primitive cultures lacked metal pots, they would often place hot stones directly into the water to raise the temperature. This method required careful handling to avoid burns and ensure that the stones were properly heated to prevent cracking.

In addition to cooking over open flames, hot stones were used extensively in various cultures worldwide as a means to prepare food. This technique, known as "stone cooking," is believed to have originated in prehistoric times and was refined over the centuries. The principle behind hot stone cooking is relatively straightforward: stones are heated in a fire and then used to cook food by either placing the food directly on the hot surface or surrounding it with heated stones.

One of the most notable examples of hot stone cooking is the use of the traditional pit oven. To prepare a meal, a pit is dug in the ground, and stones are placed at the bottom and heated in a fire. Once the stones are sufficiently hot, the food, often wrapped in leaves or placed in containers, is added to the pit. The pit is then covered with earth or additional vegetation to trap the heat. This method creates an environment similar to modern steaming, allowing food to cook slowly while retaining moisture and flavor.

Cooking with hot stones not only allowed for a more controlled cooking process but also enhanced the nutritional value of the food. The combination of steam and heat contributed to tenderizing tough cuts of meat and maximizing the flavors of vegetables and grains. This technique is particularly effective for cooking whole animals, as it allows for even cooking and prevents drying out.

In terms of nutrition, cooking with fire and hot stones offers several benefits. The Maillard reaction, a chemical reaction between amino acids and reducing sugars that occurs during cooking, enhances the flavor and aroma of food. This reaction is responsible for the appealing browned crust on roasted meats and baked goods. Furthermore, cooking increases the bioavailability of certain nutrients, such as beta-carotene in carrots and lycopene in tomatoes, making them easier for the body to absorb.

Another aspect of cooking with fire and hot stones is the communal experience it fosters. Preparing meals over an open flame or in a pit often involves gathering with family or community members, sharing stories, and collaborating in the cooking process. This communal aspect of cooking has deep cultural significance, promoting social bonds and cultural traditions that persist to this day.

Despite advances in modern cooking techniques, the methods of cooking with fire and hot stones remain relevant in contemporary culinary practices. Outdoor cooking, barbecues, and traditional earth oven techniques are popular among food enthusiasts, reflecting a desire to reconnect with the roots of human culinary heritage. The flavors produced by cooking over an open flame or using hot stones evoke a sense of nostalgia and appreciation for the simplicity and authenticity of ancient cooking practices.

Moreover, cooking with fire and hot stones can be considered a sustainable approach to food preparation. The use of natural materials and open flames minimizes reliance on processed equipment, encouraging individuals to engage directly with their environment. By sourcing local materials and utilizing traditional cooking methods, individuals can reduce their ecological footprint while embracing the rich history of human culinary practices.

In conclusion, cooking with fire and hot stones encapsulates the essence of primitive culinary techniques that have shaped human culture and nutrition for millennia. From the transformative power of fire to the ingenious use of heated stones, these methods demonstrate the remarkable adaptability and resourcefulness of our ancestors. As we explore the history and significance of cooking with fire and hot stones, we not only gain insight into our dietary heritage but also foster a deeper appreciation for the connections between food, culture, and the environment. Embracing these ancient practices allows us to honor our past while continuing to nourish ourselves in the present.

Nutritional Principles from Ancient Diets

The study of ancient diets offers invaluable insights into the nutritional principles that have sustained human life for millennia. As societies evolved, so too did their food sources, preparation methods, and dietary practices. By examining these ancient diets, we can uncover the core nutritional principles that contributed to the health and longevity of early human populations, many of which remain relevant and applicable in today's world.

At the heart of ancient dietary practices is the concept of whole foods, which encompass unprocessed or minimally processed ingredients that are close to their natural state. Early humans relied heavily on their immediate environment for sustenance, consuming a diverse array of plants, animals, and fungi. This diversity ensured a broad spectrum of nutrients, vitamins, and minerals essential for maintaining optimal health. Archaeological evidence shows that ancient peoples often foraged for wild fruits, vegetables, nuts, and seeds, which provided essential carbohydrates, healthy fats, and protein.

One of the standout nutritional principles of ancient diets is the emphasis on seasonal eating. Ancient cultures had to adapt their diets according to the seasonal availability of food. In the spring and summer, when fruits and vegetables were plentiful, they would consume large quantities of these fresh foods. In the fall and winter, preservation methods such as drying, smoking, and fermenting were employed to ensure a stable food supply. This not only allowed them to maximize nutrient intake during peak harvests but also contributed to a varied diet that reflected the natural rhythms of the earth.

Another essential principle of ancient diets is the concept of food as medicine. Many early societies understood the healing properties of certain plants and herbs, integrating them into their daily meals and medicinal practices. For instance, ancient Egyptians utilized garlic for its antiseptic properties and honey for its antibacterial effects. Similarly, traditional Chinese medicine emphasizes the role of food in maintaining health and preventing illness, advocating for a balanced diet that supports the body's natural systems.

Moreover, ancient diets were characterized by a strong connection to local ecosystems. The sourcing of food was intrinsically linked to the land, with communities relying on local flora and fauna for sustenance. This connection not only fostered a sense of stewardship for the environment but also ensured that the foods consumed were well-adapted to the individuals' nutritional needs. For example, coastal communities relied heavily on fish and marine resources, while inland tribes focused on hunting and gathering terrestrial plants and animals. This practice underscores the importance of understanding and respecting local ecosystems in contemporary dietary practices.

Protein sources in ancient diets varied significantly based on geography and available resources. While some communities depended heavily on animal protein, others thrived on plant-based diets rich in legumes, nuts, and seeds. For example, the Inuit people relied on fish, seals, and whales for protein, while many indigenous tribes in Central and South America cultivated quinoa, amaranth, and various beans. These protein sources not only provided essential amino acids but also contributed to a balanced intake of nutrients. The ancient principle of balance extended to all aspects of the diet, promoting moderation and variety.

Fats, often misunderstood in modern nutrition, were crucial components of ancient diets. The early human diet included healthy fats from sources like fish, nuts, seeds, and avocados. These fats provided essential fatty acids necessary for brain function and overall health. Moreover, ancient peoples often used animal fats in cooking, which increased the bioavailability of fat-soluble vitamins A, D, E, and K. The balance of macronutrients—carbohydrates, proteins, and fats—was a cornerstone of ancient dietary wisdom, emphasizing the need for a holistic approach to nutrition.

Another notable aspect of ancient diets is the role of fermented foods. Across cultures, fermentation was a natural preservation method that also enhanced the nutritional profile of food. Foods like yogurt, sauerkraut, and kimchi are rich in probiotics, which support gut health and immune function. The consumption of fermented foods dates back thousands of years and highlights the importance of maintaining a healthy gut microbiome, which has gained renewed attention in modern nutritional science. The principles of fermentation not only contributed to food preservation but also enriched diets with beneficial microorganisms that promoted health.

Hydration is a crucial yet often overlooked aspect of ancient nutrition. While our ancestors relied primarily on natural water sources, they also consumed hydrating foods such as fruits and vegetables. Early societies recognized the importance of water in maintaining health and wellness, often utilizing local sources to meet their hydration needs. The incorporation of broths and herbal infusions further enhanced their fluid intake, providing nourishment and hydration simultaneously.

Furthermore, the communal aspect of ancient eating practices cannot be understated. Meals were often shared experiences, fostering social bonds and reinforcing cultural traditions. Gathering for meals not only provided nourishment but also allowed for the transfer of knowledge, skills, and customs among community members. This sense of community is increasingly recognized as essential for mental and emotional well-being, emphasizing that nutrition is not just about the food itself but also about the social connections formed around it.

Incorporating the principles of ancient diets into modern eating habits can lead to improved health outcomes and a greater appreciation for the diverse foods available to us. Embracing whole foods, seasonal eating, and the consumption of fermented products can enhance our diets, providing a balance of nutrients that support overall wellness. Additionally, recognizing the importance of community and connection in the act of eating encourages us to cultivate relationships with others, sharing meals and experiences that nourish not only our bodies but also our souls.

Ultimately, the nutritional principles derived from ancient diets serve as a timeless reminder of the importance of simplicity, variety, and balance in our approach to food. By learning from the practices of our ancestors, we can cultivate healthier eating habits that align with the natural world and honor the profound relationship between food, culture, and human well-being.

Building Simple Clay or Rock Ovens

The art of cooking has evolved significantly over the centuries, yet some of the most effective and efficient methods have their roots in ancient practices. Among these, the construction and use of simple clay or rock ovens stand out as a remarkable testament to human ingenuity and adaptability. These ovens were designed to harness the power of fire, providing a reliable means for baking, roasting, and steaming food. The simplicity of their design and the materials required make them accessible to anyone looking to connect with traditional cooking methods while enhancing their culinary repertoire.

The concept of clay and rock ovens dates back thousands of years, with evidence of their use found in various cultures across the globe. From the earthen ovens of indigenous peoples to the clay tandoors of India, these ancient cooking structures demonstrate a profound understanding of thermal dynamics and efficient heat retention. By building an oven from natural materials, individuals can create a versatile cooking space that retains heat and distributes it evenly, resulting in perfectly cooked meals.

To build a simple clay or rock oven, the first step is to gather the necessary materials. Clay is often the primary component, sourced from local earth, which can be shaped and molded to form the structure of the oven. Additionally, rocks can be used to create a sturdy foundation and enhance heat retention. The type of clay used is crucial; it should be high in silica and low in organic matter to ensure durability and resistance to cracking during the heating process.

Once the materials are collected, the construction process can begin. The first step involves selecting a suitable location, ideally a flat area away from flammable materials and in close proximity to a firewood source. After clearing the area, a base is created using stones or bricks to provide stability and support for the oven structure. This base should be slightly elevated to facilitate airflow and prevent moisture from seeping into the oven.

Next, a dome shape is formed using clay. The dome is essential for capturing and retaining heat, allowing for even cooking throughout the oven. To create the dome, a form or mold can be constructed using sand or straw to support the clay until it dries. The clay is then applied in layers, ensuring that the walls are thick enough to withstand the heat without cracking. The opening of the oven should be large enough to accommodate the placement of food while also allowing for easy access.

As the clay is applied, it's essential to create a flue or chimney to allow smoke and heat to escape. This design not only prevents the buildup of smoke within the cooking chamber but also ensures an even distribution of heat. Once the structure is complete, it should be left to dry for several days, allowing the clay to harden and cure. Depending on the climate, this drying process can take longer, so patience is key.

Once the oven is fully dry, it can be fired for the first time to test its durability. A small fire is lit inside, allowing the clay to gradually heat up. This initial firing helps to solidify the structure and reveal any weaknesses that may need to be addressed. If cracks appear, they can be filled with additional clay and left to dry before conducting further tests.

The beauty of clay and rock ovens lies in their versatility. They can be used for various cooking methods, including baking bread, roasting meats, and even making pizzas. To bake bread, for example, the oven needs to be preheated for a period, allowing the walls to absorb heat. Once the desired temperature is reached, the bread can be placed inside, where it will cook evenly, developing a delicious crust and a soft interior.

Roasting meats in a clay oven is another rewarding experience. The even heat distribution allows for succulent results, as the meat cooks through while retaining moisture. Vegetables can also be roasted alongside the meat, enhancing their flavors as they absorb the smoke and heat from the oven. This method of cooking not only nourishes the body but also fosters a deeper appreciation for the ingredients and the process of creating meals from scratch.

Another popular use of clay ovens is for steaming. By placing a pot of water inside the oven alongside the food, steam can circulate, cooking the food gently and retaining its natural flavors and nutrients. This method is particularly beneficial for preparing vegetables, ensuring they remain crisp and vibrant while infused with the essence of the surrounding ingredients.

Building and using a simple clay or rock oven connects individuals to their ancestral roots and promotes a sustainable approach to cooking. By utilizing natural materials and methods, we can appreciate the art of traditional cooking while reducing our reliance on modern appliances. Moreover, the communal aspect of using an outdoor oven encourages gatherings and shared meals, fostering a sense of togetherness that is often lost in today's fast-paced society.

In conclusion, the nutritional principles derived from ancient diets and the construction of simple clay or rock ovens highlight the profound connection between food, culture, and community. By embracing these practices, individuals can nourish their bodies with wholesome, natural foods while rediscovering the joy of cooking and sharing meals with others. The wisdom of our ancestors serves as a reminder that the simplest methods can yield the most satisfying results, creating a deeper appreciation for the art of food and the experiences it brings.

Shelter Construction and Camp Building

Creating Temporary and Long-Term Shelters

The ability to construct shelters is one of humanity's fundamental survival skills, crucial for protection against the elements and for providing a safe place to rest and gather. Throughout history, various cultures have developed a myriad of shelter types, utilizing the resources available in their environment. Understanding how to create both temporary and long-term shelters is essential for anyone seeking to thrive in wilderness settings, whether for survival, exploration, or recreation.

Temporary shelters are typically designed for short-term use, often in response to immediate needs such as adverse weather conditions or unexpected circumstances. These shelters can be constructed quickly and with minimal resources, making them ideal for survival situations or outdoor excursions. One common temporary shelter is the tarp shelter, which can be made using a lightweight tarp or poncho. By securing the tarp to trees or poles with ropes, a simple overhead cover can be created to shield occupants from rain or sun.

Another effective temporary shelter is the debris hut, which utilizes natural materials like leaves, branches, and grasses. To construct a debris hut, begin by finding a sturdy branch or log, which will serve as the framework. The branch should be leaned against a tree or another sturdy object at a slight angle, creating a sloped roof. Next, a thick layer of insulation material, such as leaves or grass, is added to the frame. This layer not only provides shelter from the elements but also serves as insulation to retain heat. The entrance can be covered with additional debris to enhance protection.

In contrast, long-term shelters require more planning and construction time, as they are intended for extended stays or permanent habitation. These shelters often incorporate sturdier materials and more complex designs to provide durability and comfort. One popular long-term shelter design is the earth lodge, commonly used by indigenous peoples of North America. Earth lodges are built partially underground, providing excellent insulation against cold weather. To create an earth lodge, a circular pit is dug into the ground, followed by the construction of a wooden frame that forms the walls. The walls are then covered with a layer of earth, providing thermal mass that keeps the interior warm in winter and cool in summer.

Another effective long-term shelter is the log cabin, which utilizes logs as the primary building material. The logs are stacked horizontally, with notches cut at the ends to interlock them securely. The construction process involves laying the logs on a solid foundation and sealing the gaps with natural materials like moss or clay to improve insulation. Log cabins can be built to various sizes and styles, depending on the intended use and available resources. They provide excellent durability and can withstand harsh weather conditions.

A critical factor in both temporary and long-term shelter construction is location. Finding an appropriate site is essential for maximizing safety and comfort. Look for flat, dry ground away from potential hazards such as falling branches or flooding. Proximity to resources such as water, firewood, and foraging areas can also enhance the functionality of a shelter. Additionally, it is vital to consider the direction of prevailing winds and sunlight when positioning a shelter. Facing the entrance away from the wind can help reduce exposure to cold drafts, while maximizing sunlight exposure can aid in heating the shelter during the day.

Ventilation is another important consideration when constructing shelters, particularly in long-term designs. Proper airflow helps prevent the buildup of moisture, which can lead to mold and mildew, as well as maintain a comfortable living environment. Ventilation can be achieved through small openings or adjustable flaps in the shelter's design, allowing fresh air to circulate while keeping out rain and snow.

Assembling a shelter requires more than just physical materials; it often necessitates a blend of skills, resourcefulness, and creativity. Understanding the natural environment and utilizing available resources effectively can lead to the successful construction of functional shelters. Whether creating a simple tarp setup for an overnight camping trip or a robust earth lodge for extended habitation, the principles of shelter construction remain rooted in human ingenuity and adaptability.

Insulation and Heating Techniques

Insulation and heating techniques play a pivotal role in ensuring that shelters are not only protective but also comfortable and livable. The ability to retain heat in colder environments while allowing for proper ventilation is essential for maintaining a healthy living space. Throughout history, various cultures have developed ingenious methods to insulate and heat their shelters, using the materials available in their surroundings.

One of the simplest and most effective insulation techniques is the use of natural materials. Insulating a shelter can be achieved by filling gaps and crevices with materials such as straw, grass, leaves, or moss. These materials trap air, which serves as an insulator, preventing heat loss. For example, an earth lodge, as mentioned earlier, benefits from the thick earthen walls that provide substantial thermal mass, keeping the interior warm in winter and cool in summer. The insulation properties of natural materials extend not only to the walls but also to the roof, where a thick layer of grass or leaves can be used to minimize heat loss.

In addition to utilizing natural insulating materials, the design of the shelter itself plays a crucial role in maintaining warmth. For instance, domed structures, like those used by indigenous Arctic peoples, are highly efficient at retaining heat due to their shape. The curved surfaces reduce the amount of exposed area, minimizing heat loss and creating a cozy atmosphere inside. In contrast, structures with flat roofs or square designs can experience more heat loss, making them less effective in cold climates.

Once a shelter is adequately insulated, the focus shifts to heating techniques. The traditional method of heating a shelter involves using a fire, which can provide both warmth and light. Building a central fire pit within the shelter is a common practice, as it allows for efficient heat distribution. However, it is essential to ensure proper ventilation to prevent smoke buildup, which can be hazardous. In ancient times, many cultures built chimneys or flues to direct smoke outside while retaining warmth inside. This technique not only enhances comfort but also promotes safety.

Another effective heating technique is the use of thermal mass. This principle involves utilizing materials that can absorb, store, and gradually release heat. For example, stone or clay can be incorporated into the design of a shelter to serve as thermal mass. When heated, these materials retain warmth, gradually releasing it into the living space over time. This method helps maintain a consistent temperature within the shelter, reducing the need for continuous fires.

In regions where firewood is scarce or during long-term habitation, alternative heating methods may be employed. One such technique is the use of solar energy. By strategically placing windows or openings on the south side of a shelter, sunlight can be harnessed during the day to warm the interior. South-facing windows act as passive solar collectors, allowing sunlight to enter and warm surfaces, which then radiate heat into the space. This method requires careful planning and consideration of seasonal changes in sunlight but can significantly reduce reliance on traditional heating methods.

Heating stones can also be used as a portable option for warming a shelter. By placing stones in a fire until they are hot, they can be carefully removed and placed inside the shelter to provide radiating warmth. This technique is particularly useful in temporary shelters, as it allows for quick heating without the need for a built-in fireplace.

Another ancient method of heating shelters is the use of hot rocks, which can be heated directly in a fire and then strategically placed within the shelter to radiate heat. This technique can be particularly effective in conjunction with insulation materials, as the warm rocks will help maintain a comfortable temperature, especially during cold nights.

In summary, insulation and heating techniques are crucial components of shelter construction, significantly impacting the comfort and safety of those living within. By understanding the properties of natural materials, utilizing effective design principles, and incorporating innovative heating methods, individuals can create shelters that provide a warm and welcoming environment regardless of the external conditions. As we continue to learn from the past, these techniques remind us of the resilience and ingenuity of human beings in the face of nature's challenges. Whether building a temporary refuge for a night under the stars or a long-term home, mastering these principles can enhance our ability to thrive in the great outdoors.

Setting Up Camp for Community Living

Establishing a camp for community living involves more than merely pitching tents or setting up shelters; it requires thoughtful planning, cooperation, and consideration of the needs of all members. Historically, many cultures have understood the importance of communal living, fostering connections among individuals while ensuring shared responsibilities and resources. In today's context, whether for a short-term outdoor retreat, a survival scenario, or a long-term communal living project, the principles of effective camp setup remain crucial.

The first step in creating a successful community camp is selecting an appropriate site. This choice involves considering various factors, including access to natural resources, terrain, and safety. Ideally, the campsite should be situated near a water source for easy access, yet far enough away to avoid contamination from waste or runoff. A flat, elevated area helps prevent flooding and provides stable ground for tents or shelters. Additionally, proximity to firewood is essential for cooking and heating, making sure that these resources are abundant in the surrounding area.

Once a site is chosen, organizing the layout of the camp becomes a priority. The arrangement of shelters should foster a sense of community while providing adequate privacy for individuals or families. Common practice involves creating a central gathering area, which serves as the hub of social activity. This space can accommodate communal cooking, dining, and meetings, encouraging interaction among campers. Surrounding this common area, individual or family shelters can be positioned, allowing for a balance between communal engagement and personal space.

A communal kitchen area is an essential feature of any community camp setup. This space should be equipped with fire pits, cooking equipment, and adequate preparation surfaces. Designating a specific area for food storage and cooking helps prevent contamination and encourages hygienic practices. In traditional communities, outdoor kitchens often utilize natural materials for cooking, such as flat stones or clay for ovens. Incorporating these techniques can enhance the communal cooking experience, bringing people together in the process of food preparation and fostering a sense of shared responsibility.

In addition to a kitchen, it is vital to establish designated areas for sanitation and waste management. This is particularly important in longer-term camps where maintaining hygiene is crucial for health and wellbeing. Creating a latrine away from the camp and water sources helps minimize contamination risks. Furthermore, implementing a composting system for organic waste can contribute to sustainability and promote recycling within the community. Teaching and encouraging responsible waste management practices ensures that the environment remains clean and healthy for everyone.

Fire is a central element in community living, serving multiple purposes, from cooking and heating to providing warmth and light. Establishing a communal fire pit is not only practical but also symbolic of gathering and togetherness. It becomes a place for sharing stories, cooking meals, and creating memories. Safety measures should be in place, including clearing flammable materials from the area and having water or sand available for emergencies.

Communication and collaboration are essential aspects of camp life. Establishing roles and responsibilities within the community promotes a sense of ownership and belonging. Each member can contribute their skills to ensure the camp runs smoothly. For instance, designating individuals to handle cooking, cleaning, or maintenance tasks can help distribute the workload fairly. Regular meetings can facilitate communication and encourage members to voice their needs, concerns, and ideas for improvement.

In addition to practical considerations, fostering a sense of community spirit is paramount. Activities and events that promote bonding among campers can enhance the overall experience. Group games, communal meals, storytelling sessions, or even workshops to share skills can create lasting connections and camaraderie. These activities help break down barriers and establish trust, enabling individuals to work together harmoniously.

As the camp develops, integrating natural elements into the living space can enhance the experience. Incorporating plants, trees, and landscaping features not only beautifies the environment but also offers practical benefits. For example, creating shaded areas with trees provides relief from the sun, while herbs and edible plants can contribute to food sources. In many traditional communities, gardens serve as a vital source of sustenance, bringing individuals together in the shared labor of cultivation.

Another consideration in setting up a camp for community living is ensuring adequate access to resources for personal and communal activities. Providing designated areas for relaxation, recreation, and even creative pursuits fosters a holistic living environment. Spaces for art, music, and crafts encourage self-expression while enhancing the overall sense of community. These areas can be simple but should be thoughtfully placed to encourage participation and engagement.

Security and safety are paramount in any community setup. Establishing a system for monitoring the camp perimeter and fostering a culture of vigilance among community members ensures everyone's safety. Setting up watch duties, especially at night, can help maintain a secure environment. Creating a culture of respect and care for one another fosters a safe and nurturing atmosphere where individuals feel comfortable and supported.

As the camp evolves, embracing adaptability is key. Being flexible to changing needs and circumstances helps maintain harmony within the community. As people come and go, or as resource availability fluctuates, adapting to these changes ensures that the camp remains a vibrant and welcoming place.

In conclusion, setting up a camp for community living involves careful consideration of location, organization, sanitation, and communication. By creating a harmonious environment that fosters interaction and collaboration, individuals can experience the benefits of communal living. Embracing ancient wisdom while incorporating modern practices can lead to a fulfilling and enriching experience for all involved. In this shared space, the art of living together harmoniously is cultivated, creating a supportive community that thrives on cooperation, respect, and the joys of communal life. The skills and values developed in such settings not only enhance survival but also contribute to a deeper understanding of the connections between individuals and the natural world.

Ancient Farming and Gardening Techniques

Crop Rotation and Soil Enrichment

In ancient agricultural practices, crop rotation and soil enrichment emerged as vital techniques that significantly influenced food production and sustainability. These methods not only optimized land use but also contributed to long-term soil health and fertility, forming the cornerstone of successful farming practices across various civilizations.

Crop rotation, a method involving the systematic changing of crops planted in a specific area over time, was employed by ancient farmers to combat the depletion of soil nutrients. This practice stemmed from a profound understanding of plant biology and the natural cycles of growth. Different crops utilize and replenish different nutrients from the soil. For instance, legumes, such as peas and beans, have a unique ability to fix atmospheric nitrogen into the soil through their root nodules. This nitrogen fixation enriches the soil and provides a necessary nutrient for subsequent crops. Thus, rotating nitrogen-fixing plants with crops that require higher nitrogen levels, like grains, creates a natural fertilization cycle that enhances soil fertility.

The ancient Egyptians exemplified effective crop rotation through their practices along the Nile River. They alternated between growing wheat and barley with legumes and other crops to maintain soil health and optimize yields. This system allowed them to maximize their agricultural potential while minimizing the risk of crop failure due to nutrient depletion. Similarly, the Romans adopted crop rotation as a means to maintain the productivity of their extensive agricultural lands, implementing a three-field system. This involved rotating crops among three fields: one planted with grains, another with legumes, and the third left fallow. This method not only prevented soil exhaustion but also provided ample time for natural replenishment.

Another essential aspect of ancient crop rotation practices was the integration of fallow periods. Leaving a field fallow for a season allowed it to rest and recover, during which time natural processes enriched the soil. During this period, weeds and other plants could grow, contributing organic matter to the soil when they decomposed. This practice helped restore nutrient levels and prevent soil erosion, fostering a healthier agricultural environment.

Soil enrichment techniques were equally important in ancient farming. Cultivators recognized the necessity of maintaining soil structure, fertility, and moisture retention to support healthy crop growth. Various methods were employed to enrich the soil, including the incorporation of organic matter, composting, and the use of natural fertilizers. Ancient farmers often relied on animal manure, composted plant materials, and even ash from burned plants to enhance soil fertility. These organic amendments improved soil texture, increased moisture retention, and provided a steady supply of essential nutrients.

In many cultures, the practice of intercropping—planting different crops in proximity—was common. This method maximized the use of space and resources while promoting soil health. For example, the traditional practice of planting maize, beans, and squash together, known as the "Three Sisters," exemplifies the benefits of intercropping. Each crop serves a unique purpose:

maize provides support for the climbing beans, beans fix nitrogen in the soil, and squash spreads out, shading the ground and preventing weeds. This harmonious relationship among the plants not only boosts crop yields but also enhances soil fertility.

In addition to these practices, ancient farmers often utilized natural landscape features to their advantage. They understood the importance of topography, water availability, and microclimates in determining the best locations for various crops. Terracing, for example, was a technique used by ancient civilizations in mountainous regions, allowing them to cultivate sloped areas effectively. This method reduced soil erosion, enhanced water retention, and created microclimates that benefited certain crops.

As agricultural practices evolved, the wisdom of crop rotation and soil enrichment remained foundational principles that guided farmers in their quest for sustainability and productivity. The understanding of soil as a living ecosystem, capable of supporting diverse plant life, was intrinsic to many ancient cultures. This holistic approach to agriculture not only addressed the immediate needs of food production but also recognized the importance of maintaining the health of the land for future generations.

Today, modern agriculture continues to draw inspiration from these ancient practices. The growing awareness of the need for sustainable farming methods has led to a resurgence of interest in crop rotation and soil enrichment. Many contemporary farmers are adopting organic farming techniques that echo the principles established by their ancestors, recognizing that healthy soil is the key to productive crops.

In conclusion, crop rotation and soil enrichment were critical elements of ancient farming techniques that laid the groundwork for sustainable agricultural practices. By understanding the interrelationships between crops, soil health, and the environment, ancient farmers created systems that maximized productivity while ensuring the longevity of their land. These time-tested principles continue to inform modern agricultural practices, reminding us of the enduring value of ancient wisdom in fostering a sustainable future. As we look toward addressing contemporary challenges in food production and environmental stewardship, the lessons learned from our ancestors can guide us in cultivating a more resilient and sustainable agricultural landscape.

Companion Planting for Enhanced Yields

Companion planting, a time-honored agricultural technique practiced by ancient civilizations, involves the strategic placement of different plant species in proximity to one another to promote mutual benefits. This method not only enhances plant health and productivity but also fosters a balanced ecosystem within the garden or farm. By understanding the natural relationships between plants, ancient farmers cultivated diverse crops that thrived in harmony, ultimately leading to increased yields and sustainable agricultural practices.

The principles of companion planting are rooted in the observation of nature and the interactions between various plant species. Ancient farmers recognized that certain plants possess qualities that can either enhance or inhibit the growth of their neighbors. By intentionally pairing compatible plants, they were able to maximize the use of space, optimize resource sharing, and deter pests. For instance, many indigenous cultures relied on specific plant combinations to bolster crop yields while minimizing the need for chemical inputs.

One of the most renowned examples of companion planting is the Three Sisters method practiced by Native American tribes. This technique involves the intercropping of maize (corn), beans, and squash, which work synergistically to create a thriving garden. The tall maize provides a natural trellis for the climbing beans, while the beans, as nitrogen-fixing plants, enrich the soil with vital nutrients. Meanwhile, the sprawling squash plants cover the ground, suppressing weeds and retaining soil moisture. This intricate relationship not only maximizes space but also enhances the overall health of the garden, demonstrating the profound understanding that ancient farmers had of plant interactions.

Companion planting extends beyond simply planting compatible species together; it also incorporates the notion of biodiversity. By cultivating a diverse range of plants, ancient farmers created resilient ecosystems that could withstand pests and diseases. For example, planting aromatic herbs, such as basil or marigold, alongside vegetable crops can repel harmful insects, acting as a natural pest deterrent. The scent of these companion plants masks the aroma of the vegetables, confusing pests and reducing their impact on the main crops. This method of natural pest control allowed ancient farmers to maintain healthy crops without the use of synthetic pesticides.

Moreover, the benefits of companion planting extend to soil health as well. Certain plants, like deep-rooted perennials, can improve soil structure and nutrient availability. When paired with shallow-rooted annuals, they create a symbiotic relationship that promotes efficient resource utilization. For instance, radishes, which have a quick growth cycle, can be sown alongside slower-growing crops like carrots. The radishes germinate and mature quickly, breaking up the soil while leaving space for the carrots to develop, resulting in enhanced yields for both crops.

In addition to nutrient sharing and pest management, companion planting fosters improved pollination. By introducing flowering plants that attract beneficial insects, such as bees and butterflies, ancient farmers could increase pollination rates in their crops. For instance, planting flowers like calendula or borage among vegetable crops not only enhances the aesthetic appeal of the garden but also encourages pollinators to visit, resulting in more abundant fruit and seed production.

Ancient agricultural societies also understood the importance of timing when implementing companion planting strategies. They would plant crops according to seasonal cycles and lunar phases, ensuring that each plant received the optimal conditions for growth. This holistic approach reflects a deep connection with the natural rhythms of the environment and highlights the importance of understanding the unique requirements of each species.

The legacy of companion planting continues to influence modern agricultural practices. As awareness of the detrimental effects of monoculture and chemical inputs grows, many contemporary farmers and gardeners are embracing the wisdom of ancient practices. Organic and permaculture movements advocate for the use of companion planting as a means of promoting biodiversity, enhancing soil health, and reducing pest pressures. By implementing these time-tested techniques, modern cultivators can work in harmony with nature, ensuring sustainable food production for future generations.

Furthermore, companion planting fosters a deeper understanding of the interconnectedness of plants and the ecosystems they inhabit. It encourages gardeners to become more attuned to their environment, promoting observation and experimentation. By observing how different plants interact and respond to various conditions, individuals can develop a more nuanced understanding of their local ecosystem, leading to more effective gardening practices.

In conclusion, companion planting represents a fundamental aspect of ancient agricultural wisdom that continues to offer valuable insights for modern cultivation. By recognizing and harnessing the natural relationships between plants, ancient farmers achieved enhanced yields, improved pest management, and healthier soils. The principles of companion planting emphasize the importance of biodiversity and ecological balance in agriculture, highlighting the need for sustainable practices that benefit both the environment and food production. As we navigate the challenges of contemporary agriculture, embracing the lessons learned from our ancestors can guide us toward more resilient and sustainable farming practices, ensuring food security and environmental stewardship for generations to come. Through the art of companion planting, we can cultivate not only productive gardens but also a deeper appreciation for the interconnectedness of life in our ecosystems.

Seed saving and cultivating native plants are practices deeply rooted in ancient agricultural traditions. These techniques not only promote biodiversity and ecological balance but also empower communities to sustain themselves through a self-sufficient approach to food production. By understanding the significance of these practices, we can appreciate their role in fostering resilience in ecosystems and food systems.

Seed saving is the process of collecting and preserving seeds from plants to be replanted in subsequent seasons. This ancient practice has been essential for ensuring food security and preserving genetic diversity in crops. Early agricultural societies recognized that seeds from well-adapted plants would yield crops best suited to their local environment. By saving seeds from the most vigorous and resilient plants, ancient farmers could gradually select for traits that suited their specific growing conditions, leading to the development of local varieties that thrived over generations.

This method of cultivation also allowed communities to become less reliant on external seed sources, fostering a sense of independence and self-sufficiency. In many cultures, the practice of seed saving was not just a practical necessity but also a communal activity, fostering social ties and shared knowledge among farmers. Families would often exchange seeds, ensuring a diverse gene pool and the preservation of traditional varieties that were well adapted to local climates and soils.

Cultivating native plants is another vital aspect of sustainable agriculture that has roots in ancient practices. Native plants, which are species that naturally

143

occur in a specific region, play a crucial role in maintaining local ecosystems. They are adapted to local soil, climate, and wildlife, making them more resilient and less demanding in terms of resources compared to non-native species. By cultivating native plants, ancient farmers supported the local biodiversity and created habitats for beneficial insects, pollinators, and wildlife.

The importance of native plants extends beyond ecological benefits; they also hold cultural significance for many communities. Indigenous peoples often cultivated native plants not only for food but also for medicinal purposes, ceremonial practices, and as sources of materials for crafts. For example, the cultivation of traditional crops like maize, squash, and beans by Native American tribes was integral to their cultural identity and survival. These crops, often referred to as the "Three Sisters," were grown together to maximize yields and support one another's growth. The practices surrounding these crops were deeply embedded in their cultural traditions and worldview.

The practice of seed saving and the cultivation of native plants align seamlessly with the principles of permaculture and agroecology, which emphasize working with nature rather than against it. These approaches encourage farmers and gardeners to design systems that mimic natural ecosystems, fostering biodiversity and soil health. By integrating native plants into agricultural landscapes, practitioners can create polycultures that enhance resilience and productivity while reducing the need for synthetic fertilizers and pesticides.

Moreover, the preservation of native seeds is crucial for adapting to changing environmental conditions. As climate change poses new challenges to agriculture, the genetic diversity inherent in traditional seed varieties becomes invaluable. These local varieties often possess traits that allow them to thrive in fluctuating climates, such as drought resistance or disease tolerance. By prioritizing seed saving, communities can safeguard their agricultural heritage and ensure access to crops that will adapt to future conditions.

Seed saving and cultivating native plants also play a significant role in the broader context of sustainability and environmental conservation. As industrial agriculture has spread, the reliance on a limited number of high-yield crop varieties has led to a decline in biodiversity. This monoculture system makes ecosystems more vulnerable to pests, diseases, and changing climate conditions. By shifting towards seed saving and native plant cultivation, we can actively contribute to restoring biodiversity and promoting healthier ecosystems.

In modern contexts, community seed banks and local initiatives focused on preserving traditional seed varieties have emerged in response to the need for sustainable agricultural practices. These initiatives not only empower communities to reclaim control over their food systems but also serve as repositories of cultural heritage and knowledge. By participating in seed saving efforts, individuals can connect with their agricultural roots and contribute to a global movement for food sovereignty and environmental sustainability.

In conclusion, seed saving and cultivating native plants are fundamental practices that reflect the wisdom of ancient agricultural traditions. By preserving local seed varieties and nurturing native ecosystems, communities can enhance their resilience, promote biodiversity, and foster self-sufficiency. These practices not only support sustainable agriculture but also reconnect us with our cultural heritage and the intricate relationships we share with the natural world. As we face contemporary challenges in food production and environmental degradation, embracing these ancient techniques can guide us toward a more sustainable and equitable future. Through the act of saving seeds and cultivating native plants, we can honor the legacy of our ancestors while nurturing the health of our planet for generations to come.

Navigating and Communicating in the Wilderness

Tanning Animal Hides for Clothing

Tanning animal hides is an ancient craft that transforms raw animal skins into durable materials suitable for clothing, shelter, and various other uses. This process has been practiced for millennia by cultures around the world, providing not only warmth and protection but also a connection to the environment and the animals that inhabit it. The methods of tanning have evolved over time, yet the core principles remain deeply rooted in traditional practices that highlight resourcefulness, sustainability, and a profound understanding of animal biology.

The first step in the tanning process is the careful preparation of the animal hide. Typically, this begins immediately after the animal has been harvested, as prompt skinning helps prevent spoilage. The hide is carefully removed, ensuring that it is as intact as possible. The removal of excess flesh, fat, and hair is crucial, as these elements can complicate the tanning process and affect the quality of the final product. Many ancient cultures used simple tools, such as stone scrapers or sharp bones, to meticulously clean the hide, a practice that required skill and patience.

Once the hide is prepared, the next stage involves curing to prevent decomposition. Curing methods vary across cultures but typically include salting, drying, or using smoke. Salting is one of the most common techniques, where coarse salt is rubbed into the hide to draw out moisture, effectively preserving it. Ancient peoples understood that moisture is the primary enemy of hide preservation, and the use of salt not only prevents decay but also prepares the hide for further tanning processes.

The tanning process itself is where the transformation truly occurs. Ancient tanning techniques primarily utilized natural materials, such as plant tannins, animal brains, or fats. One of the most traditional methods involves soaking the hides in a solution made from tree bark, leaves, or nuts that contain tannins, which are natural compounds that bond with the collagen fibers in the hide. This process not only preserves the hide but also makes it more flexible and resistant to water.

For example, the bark of oak trees is rich in tannins and has been widely used in traditional tanning. After being stripped from the tree, the bark is crushed and soaked in water to create a tannin-rich solution. The hide is then submerged in this solution for several days or weeks, depending on the desired final texture. This slow, methodical approach ensures that the tannins penetrate deeply into the hide, resulting in a durable and pliable material.

Another ancient technique involves using animal brains, which are rich in fats and oils. The hide is worked with the brains to facilitate the absorption of these fats, which not only preserves the hide but also imparts a soft, supple quality. This method is particularly valued in cultures where maintaining the natural softness of the hide is essential, such as in the making of clothing.

Once the tanning is complete, the hides are often dyed using natural pigments derived from plants, minerals, or insects. These dyes not only enhance the aesthetic appeal of the clothing but also serve to further protect the hides from environmental elements. The final step involves stretching and drying the hide, which helps to maintain its shape and ensures it is ready for use.

Tanned hides can be fashioned into a variety of clothing items, including garments, shoes, and accessories. The cultural significance of these creations cannot be overstated, as they often reflect the identity, status, and creativity of the communities that produced them. The art of tanning hides is not merely a functional skill; it embodies a deep-seated connection between people and nature, where every stitch tells a story of survival, adaptation, and respect for the environment.

Today, while modern methods of leather production dominate, there is a renewed interest in traditional tanning practices. Craft enthusiasts and sustainable fashion advocates are increasingly drawn to the beauty and uniqueness of hand-tanned hides. This resurgence not only preserves ancient skills but also encourages a more sustainable approach to clothing production, as it emphasizes the use of local materials and resources.

Basic Weaving and Basketry

Weaving and basketry are two ancient crafts that have served humanity for thousands of years, providing essential tools for storage, transport, and clothing. These practices showcase the creativity, resourcefulness, and craftsmanship of cultures across the globe. By using readily available natural materials, such as grasses, reeds, fibers, and animal sinew, ancient peoples developed intricate techniques to create functional and aesthetically pleasing items. The knowledge and skills associated with weaving and basketry were often passed down through generations, preserving cultural heritage and fostering community bonds.

The process of weaving involves interlacing threads or fibers to create fabric or textiles. In ancient times, weaving was primarily done using natural materials such as cotton, linen, wool, and silk. Each of these materials offered unique properties and textures, allowing for a wide range of applications. For instance, linen, derived from flax plants, was highly valued in ancient Egypt for its durability and breathability, making it ideal for clothing in warm climates.

Basic weaving can be accomplished using a simple loom, which is a device that holds the threads in place while the weaver interlaces additional threads. In its most basic form, a loom consists of two horizontal bars, one for the warp threads and another for the weft threads. The warp threads are stretched tightly across the loom, and the weaver then passes the weft threads over and under the warp threads, creating a woven fabric. This process requires skill and precision, as the tension and arrangement of the threads determine the quality of the final product.

Ancient cultures often developed unique weaving patterns and designs that reflected their environment, beliefs, and social structures. For instance, the Navajo people of the American Southwest are renowned for their intricate woven rugs, which incorporate vibrant colors and geometric patterns that hold cultural significance. These designs often tell stories or symbolize elements of their spirituality, showcasing the deep connection between their weaving practices and their cultural identity.

Basketry, on the other hand, focuses on creating containers by weaving together flexible materials such as grasses, reeds, or willow branches. The process of making a basket involves several steps, including gathering materials, preparing them for weaving, and constructing the basket itself. Traditionally, basket makers would select specific plants based on their flexibility, strength, and availability. For example, river reeds and cattails are often used for their pliability, while more rigid materials like twigs are employed for the structural framework.

Basketry techniques can vary significantly depending on the region and available materials. In some cultures, coiling is a common method, where materials are spiraled around a central point and stitched together. This technique creates strong, durable baskets that can hold a variety of items, from food to tools. In contrast, some cultures employ twining, where two or more strands are woven together in a pattern to create a fabric-like texture. This method allows for greater intricacy and creativity in design.

The use of natural dyes to color woven and basketry items further enhances their visual appeal. Many ancient cultures relied on plant-based dyes derived from roots, leaves, and berries to achieve a wide range of colors. These dyes not only added beauty but also held cultural significance, with specific colors representing different meanings or values within a community.

Both weaving and basketry served functional purposes in ancient societies, providing containers for storage, transport, and food preparation. In many cases, these crafts were essential for daily life, enabling people to carry and store food, water, and tools efficiently. Beyond their practical applications, woven and basketry items often held social and spiritual significance. For example, ceremonial baskets were often crafted for rituals or celebrations, showcasing the artistry and skill of the maker while honoring cultural traditions.

Today, weaving and basketry remain vital practices, celebrated for their artistic expression and cultural heritage. Many contemporary artisans and crafters have revitalized these ancient skills, producing both functional and decorative items that pay homage to traditional techniques. The resurgence of interest in handmade crafts has sparked a movement toward sustainability, encouraging individuals to value locally sourced materials and the time-honored skills of weaving and basketry.

In conclusion, the crafting of clothing through tanning animal hides, the art of weaving, and the intricate practice of basketry exemplify the resourcefulness and creativity of ancient cultures. These practices not only provided essential tools and garments for survival but also served as a means of cultural expression and identity. By understanding and appreciating the significance of these crafts, we can connect with our ancestral roots and honor the traditions that have shaped human societies for millennia. Embracing these ancient techniques today not only fosters sustainability and creativity but also reinforces our connection to the natural world and the communities that have thrived alongside it.

Stone and Bone Tool Crafting

Stone and bone tool crafting is one of the oldest forms of technology developed by human beings, tracing back to prehistoric times. This ancient practice involved the creation of tools and weapons from readily available materials found in the environment, showcasing the ingenuity and adaptability of our ancestors. By understanding the methods and significance of stone and bone tool crafting, we can gain insights into the survival strategies and cultural practices of ancient communities.

The crafting of stone tools began with the use of percussion techniques, where one rock was struck against another to create sharp edges. This process, known as knapping, enabled early humans to fashion tools such as hand axes, scrapers, and projectile points. The choice of stone was critical, with materials like flint, obsidian, and chert being favored for their ability to be shaped and honed into cutting edges. The skill of knapping required practice and knowledge of the properties of different stones, as well as an understanding of the desired shape and function of the tool.

One of the most significant advancements in stone tool technology was the development of the bifacial technique, where both sides of the tool were shaped to create a sharper edge. This technique allowed for more efficient and versatile tools that could be used for various tasks, such as hunting, butchering, and woodworking. Bifacial tools were often used in conjunction with other materials, such as wood or bone, to create composite tools that enhanced their functionality.

Bone tools also played a crucial role in the lives of ancient peoples, especially in regions where stone was scarce. Bones from hunted animals were shaped and sharpened to create tools such as awls, needles, and fish hooks. The crafting of bone tools involved careful planning and skill, as the bone had to be properly cleaned, dried, and shaped. Often, the marrow was extracted for food, leaving behind a hollow tube that could be further fashioned into tools.

In some cultures, the artistic aspects of stone and bone tool crafting were just as important as their functional uses. Tools and weapons were often adorned with carvings or decorations, reflecting the beliefs and values of the community. The craftsmanship involved in creating these tools fostered a sense of identity and connection among the makers, reinforcing their relationship with their environment and the resources it provided.

The techniques of stone and bone tool crafting were not static; they evolved over time as societies developed and adapted to changing conditions. As human populations grew and migrated, the exchange of knowledge and materials facilitated innovation in tool-making practices. The advent of metallurgy marked a significant turning point in this evolution, as the ability to work with metals allowed for even greater advancements in tool and weapon design.

Despite the shift to metal tools, the principles of stone and bone tool crafting remain relevant today, especially in the context of survival skills and self-sufficiency. Many modern survivalists and enthusiasts seek to revive these ancient techniques, recognizing their practicality and effectiveness in outdoor settings. Workshops and classes on flint knapping and bone tool making have gained popularity, providing individuals with hands-on experiences in ancient craftsmanship.

Furthermore, the sustainable nature of stone and bone tool crafting aligns with contemporary values of environmental stewardship and resource conservation. By utilizing natural materials and practicing traditional techniques, individuals can develop a deeper appreciation for their connection to the earth and the resources it offers. This awareness fosters a sense of responsibility toward the environment and encourages sustainable practices in modern living.

In conclusion, the crafting and maintenance of basic clothing and gear through the tanning of animal hides, basic weaving, basketry, and stone and bone tool crafting reflect the ingenuity and resourcefulness of ancient cultures. These practices not only served practical purposes for survival but also held cultural significance, fostering a sense of identity and community. By embracing and revitalizing these ancient skills, we can connect with our ancestral heritage, cultivate self-sufficiency, and promote sustainable living in a modern context. The lessons learned from these crafts continue to resonate, reminding us of the timeless wisdom embedded in our relationship with nature.

Navigating and Communicating in the Wilderness

Navigating and communicating in the wilderness has always been a crucial aspect of survival for ancient peoples. As they traversed varied landscapes and encountered challenges, they relied on their knowledge of the environment, natural phenomena, and social dynamics to thrive. Ancient signaling and communication methods, natural navigation skills, and the importance of community and group survival were essential elements of their survival strategies, ensuring safety and resourcefulness in the face of adversity.

Ancient Signaling and Communication Methods

In the absence of modern technology, ancient cultures developed ingenious methods of signaling and communication to convey important information across distances. These methods were deeply rooted in the understanding of the environment and the behaviors of animals, as well as the social structures of communities.

One of the most common forms of communication was through visual signals, which could be seen from afar. For instance, smoke signals were widely used by many Indigenous peoples across North America. By building a fire and creating smoke, they could send messages over long distances. The color, density, and duration of the smoke conveyed specific meanings, alerting others to everything from danger to the gathering of tribes. The ability to interpret and create these signals required a shared understanding among community members, showcasing the importance of communication within social groups.

Another form of visual signaling involved the use of mirrors or shiny objects to reflect sunlight. This method, often used by military forces, allowed for messages to be sent across vast expanses without the need for vocal communication. In addition to visual cues, ancient peoples also relied on sound-based signals, such as drums, horns, or whistles. These sounds could carry over long distances, alerting individuals to gatherings, warnings of danger, or the approach of a hunting party.

Additionally, the use of symbols and markings on trees or rocks served as a method of communication for tracking movements, marking territory, or conveying information about resources. Carvings, painted symbols, or specific arrangements of stones acted as a language of sorts, telling stories of the land and its inhabitants.

In many communities, storytelling was another vital aspect of communication. Oral traditions passed down knowledge about the environment, navigation techniques, and survival skills. Stories often contained lessons, warnings, and shared histories, reinforcing social bonds and ensuring that essential information was retained across generations.

Natural Navigation Skills and Mapping Techniques

Natural navigation skills are a critical component of wilderness survival, enabling individuals to find their way through unfamiliar terrain without modern tools. Ancient peoples honed their navigation abilities through keen observation of their surroundings, developing a deep understanding of natural indicators that guided their paths.

One fundamental skill in natural navigation is the ability to read the sun and stars. During the day, the sun's position in the sky indicates cardinal directions. For instance, in the Northern Hemisphere, the sun rises in the east and sets in the west. By observing the angle of the sun at different times of the day, navigators can approximate their orientation. Similarly, at night, ancient navigators relied on the stars for direction. The North Star, for example, is a fixed point in the sky that has historically served as a reliable reference for determining true north.

Landmarks also play a significant role in navigation. Ancient peoples would often memorize distinctive geographical features such as mountains, rivers, and unique rock formations. These landmarks served as natural maps, providing a frame of reference for their journeys. In addition to physical landmarks, weather patterns, animal behaviors, and the growth of vegetation also offered clues about direction and proximity to water sources or safe havens.

In some cultures, oral mapping traditions emerged, where navigators would memorize routes and share them through storytelling. These maps of knowledge often included details about resources, potential dangers, and seasonal changes in the landscape. The ability to convey and retain this information was critical for survival, as it helped communities navigate vast territories effectively.

In ancient times, survival in the wilderness was often a collective effort, underscoring the significance of community and group dynamics. Working together not only enhanced the chances of survival but also fostered social cohesion and a shared sense of purpose.

Communal living meant that resources could be pooled, and tasks could be divided among group members. For instance, while some individuals might focus on hunting, others could gather food, build shelters, or care for children. This division of labor allowed communities to thrive, as everyone contributed their unique skills and strengths.

Moreover, social bonds formed within these communities created support networks that were vital during times of crisis. In a wilderness setting, the challenges of securing food, water, and shelter could be daunting. However, with a strong sense of community, individuals could rely on one another for assistance, sharing knowledge and resources to navigate difficult situations.

Additionally, shared experiences fostered a collective knowledge base, where skills and survival techniques were passed down through generations. This transmission of knowledge was crucial for the continuity of cultural practices, ensuring that younger members of the community learned the skills necessary for survival in their specific environment.

The importance of communication within communities also cannot be overstated. Clear and effective communication was essential for coordinating group activities, from hunting expeditions to building shelters. Signals, both visual and auditory, facilitated collaboration and ensured that everyone was aware of their roles and responsibilities.

Furthermore, a strong community bond enhanced morale and psychological resilience. Facing the uncertainties of the wilderness can be isolating and challenging; however, knowing that one is part of a supportive group can provide comfort and motivation. Ancient peoples often celebrated communal achievements through rituals and gatherings, reinforcing their social connections and fostering a sense of identity and belonging.

In conclusion, navigating and communicating in the wilderness involved a rich tapestry of ancient practices that underscored the importance of community, knowledge, and adaptability. From signaling and communication methods to natural navigation skills and the collaborative nature of group survival, these elements formed the foundation of resilience in the face of challenges. As we explore the lessons of the past, we can draw inspiration from these ancient practices to cultivate a deeper appreciation for our environment and foster strong connections within our communities. Embracing the wisdom of our ancestors allows us to navigate the complexities of modern life while honoring the timeless lessons embedded in our relationship with nature and each other.

The Philosophy of Survival and Self-Reliance

The philosophy of survival and self-reliance is deeply woven into the fabric of human history, with ancient societies offering profound insights into resilience, spirituality, and the quest for fulfillment through self-sufficiency. As people faced the challenges of their environments, they developed philosophies that emphasized the importance of adaptability, inner strength, and a deep connection to nature. By examining these philosophies, we can glean valuable lessons that resonate with modern life, inspiring us to cultivate resilience, embrace spiritual practices, and pursue self-sufficiency as a means of achieving freedom and fulfillment.

Lessons from Ancient Societies on Resilience

Resilience is a central tenet of survival, and ancient societies exemplified this quality in myriad ways. The ability to withstand adversity and recover from hardships was essential for the survival of these communities. From the harsh climates of the Arctic to the arid deserts of Africa, ancient peoples developed innovative strategies to adapt to their environments, demonstrating resilience in the face of challenges.

One of the most significant lessons from ancient societies is the importance of resourcefulness. In the absence of modern conveniences, people relied on their ingenuity to make the most of what was available to them. For instance, nomadic tribes learned to use every part of an animal they hunted, from meat and hides to bones and sinew, ensuring nothing went to waste. This resourcefulness extended to plant life as well; ancient foragers identified

161

edible plants, medicinal herbs, and other resources, developing a comprehensive understanding of their environment.

Moreover, ancient societies understood the value of community in fostering resilience. Working together allowed individuals to share resources, skills, and knowledge. This collective approach strengthened social bonds and created a support network that enhanced the group's ability to cope with external challenges. Rituals and traditions played a critical role in maintaining social cohesion, providing individuals with a sense of belonging and purpose.

The stories of survival from ancient cultures often revolve around overcoming hardships through perseverance and collaboration. These narratives serve as powerful reminders that resilience is not solely an individual trait but a communal strength. By drawing on the experiences of those who came before us, we can learn to cultivate our resilience and support one another in our own journeys.

The Role of Spiritual Practices in Survival

Spirituality has always played a significant role in the lives of ancient societies, influencing their perspectives on survival and self-reliance. Spiritual practices often provided individuals with a sense of purpose, connection to the natural world, and comfort in times of uncertainty. The belief in a higher power or the interconnectedness of all living beings served as a guiding force, helping individuals navigate the challenges of life.

Many ancient cultures engaged in rituals that honored the earth, the seasons, and the cycles of life. These practices fostered a deep respect for nature and an understanding of the reciprocal relationship between humans and the environment. For instance, agricultural societies often celebrated harvest festivals, expressing gratitude for the bounty of the earth and acknowledging the importance of sustainable practices. This spiritual connection to the land instilled a sense of responsibility and stewardship, reinforcing the idea that survival depends on the health of the ecosystem.

Furthermore, spiritual practices often provided individuals with coping mechanisms during difficult times. Rituals, meditation, and prayer offered solace and a way to process emotions, helping individuals maintain a sense of inner peace amidst external chaos. The practice of mindfulness, which has roots in ancient traditions, encourages individuals to stay present and grounded, fostering resilience and emotional well-being.

In addition to personal spiritual practices, communal rituals served to strengthen social ties and foster a shared identity. When communities came together to celebrate, mourn, or seek guidance, they reinforced their bonds and collectively acknowledged the challenges they faced. This communal aspect of spirituality not only provided support but also encouraged a sense of purpose and belonging, crucial elements for survival.

Self-Sufficiency as a Path to Freedom and Fulfillment

The pursuit of self-sufficiency is an ancient philosophy that emphasizes independence, resourcefulness, and a deep connection to one's environment. For many ancient societies, self-sufficiency was not merely a means of survival; it was a path to freedom and fulfillment. The ability to provide for oneself and one's community created a sense of agency, allowing individuals to live in harmony with nature and cultivate a sustainable lifestyle.

Self-sufficiency involves a profound understanding of one's resources, whether they be natural, social, or personal. Ancient peoples developed skills in agriculture, hunting, gathering, and crafting, ensuring they could meet their basic needs without relying on external systems. This independence fostered a sense of empowerment, as individuals learned to navigate their environments and make informed choices about their sustenance.

Moreover, self-sufficiency promotes a holistic view of well-being. When individuals engage in activities such as gardening, foraging, or crafting, they connect with the rhythms of nature and develop a greater appreciation for the resources around them. This connection fosters mindfulness and encourages individuals to slow down and engage with the world in a more meaningful way. In contrast to the fast-paced, consumer-driven lifestyle of modern society, self-sufficiency invites individuals to cultivate a deeper sense of fulfillment through intentional living.

The concept of self-sufficiency also extends to emotional and spiritual well-being. By developing a strong sense of self and a connection to one's values and beliefs, individuals can navigate life's challenges with greater resilience. The wisdom of ancient societies reminds us that true fulfillment comes from within, and that self-reliance is not solely about physical survival but also about nurturing one's spirit and sense of purpose.

In today's context, the philosophy of survival and self-reliance remains relevant as we face an increasingly complex and interconnected world. The lessons from ancient societies on resilience, the role of spirituality, and the pursuit of self-sufficiency provide us with valuable tools for navigating our own challenges. By embracing these philosophies, we can cultivate a deeper connection to ourselves, our communities, and the natural world, fostering a sense of empowerment and fulfillment that transcends the material aspects of life.

In conclusion, the philosophy of survival and self-reliance offers timeless wisdom that continues to resonate with modern individuals seeking to navigate the complexities of life. By learning from ancient societies, we can cultivate resilience, honor our spiritual practices, and embrace self-sufficiency as a pathway to freedom and fulfillment. As we reconnect with these principles, we empower ourselves to thrive in an ever-changing world, drawing strength from our past while forging a meaningful path forward.

Conclusion: Adapting Ancient Skills for Modern Challenges

In an age characterized by rapid technological advancement and urbanization, the skills and wisdom of our ancestors offer invaluable insights for navigating contemporary challenges. As we confront issues like climate change, food security, and social disconnection, adapting ancient skills can empower individuals and communities to develop sustainable solutions. The wisdom of the past serves as a guide, illuminating pathways toward resilience, self-sufficiency, and a deeper connection with nature.

Applying Ancient Wisdom in a Modern Context

The principles of ancient survival skills are remarkably adaptable to modern contexts. For instance, the practice of foraging for wild edibles—once a necessity for survival—is experiencing a resurgence among those seeking to reconnect with nature and reduce their reliance on commercial food sources. By learning to identify and harvest wild plants, individuals can supplement their diets with nutritious options while fostering a deeper appreciation for local ecosystems.

Similarly, traditional farming techniques, such as crop rotation and companion planting, are gaining recognition for their environmental benefits. These practices, which prioritize soil health and biodiversity, align perfectly with contemporary sustainable agriculture movements. By incorporating ancient farming wisdom, modern farmers can improve their yields while minimizing the ecological impact of their operations.

166

Moreover, ancient building techniques, such as using natural materials for shelter construction, offer sustainable alternatives to modern construction practices. As we face a housing crisis and escalating environmental concerns, looking to the past for guidance can inspire innovative approaches to building that prioritize sustainability and community resilience.

Essential Mindsets for Sustainable Survival

To truly adapt ancient skills for modern challenges, cultivating a mindset that values sustainability, resilience, and interconnectedness is essential. This mindset encourages individuals to recognize the intricate relationships between their actions and the environment. Embracing sustainability means understanding that every choice we make—whether in our consumption habits, resource management, or lifestyle—has far-reaching consequences.

Resilience is another critical mindset to foster. Life is inherently unpredictable, and developing the ability to adapt to changing circumstances is vital for survival. By learning from ancient societies that thrived in adversity, we can cultivate a resilient spirit that embraces challenges as opportunities for growth and learning. This mindset can be nurtured through practices such as mindfulness, problem-solving, and community collaboration, empowering individuals to face uncertainty with confidence.

Additionally, recognizing the interconnectedness of all living beings fosters a sense of responsibility and stewardship for the planet. Ancient cultures often viewed themselves as part of a larger web of life, understanding that their well-being was intrinsically linked to the health of their environment. By adopting this perspective, modern individuals can foster a greater sense of purpose and agency, motivating them to make choices that benefit not only themselves but also their communities and the planet as a whole.

Creating a Survival Kit with Ancient Essentials

Incorporating ancient wisdom into modern survival practices can be as simple as creating a survival kit that reflects time-tested techniques and tools. This kit can be tailored to individual needs and environments, serving as a valuable resource for emergencies, outdoor adventures, or self-sufficiency endeavors.

Essential items for a survival kit inspired by ancient practices may include:

1. **Natural Cordage**: Learning to make cordage from plant fibers or animal sinew can be invaluable for constructing shelters, traps, or tools. Incorporating this skill into a survival kit ensures preparedness for a variety of situations.

2. **Foraging Guide**: A resource for identifying edible plants, medicinal herbs, and poisonous species is essential for anyone interested in foraging. This guide can help individuals navigate their surroundings safely and effectively.

3. **Fire-Starting Tools**: Fire is a fundamental survival skill. Including traditional fire-starting tools, such as a fire drill or flint and steel, in a survival kit promotes self-sufficiency while honoring ancient methods.

4. **Basic Tool-Making Materials**: Including materials for crafting basic tools—such as stones for cutting or bones for shaping—can empower individuals to create what they need from their environment.

5. **Seeds for Native Plants**: Incorporating seeds for local edible plants into a survival kit fosters a connection to the land and promotes sustainable gardening practices.

6. **Natural First Aid Supplies**: A collection of medicinal herbs, salves, and poultices can provide essential first aid options, honoring the traditional healing practices of ancient cultures.

7. **Water Purification Methods**: Including knowledge or tools for purifying water—such as charcoal or clay pots—ensures access to safe drinking water in emergencies.

By integrating these elements into a survival kit, individuals can draw on the wisdom of the past while equipping themselves to face modern challenges.

In conclusion, the relevance of ancient skills and philosophies in today's world cannot be overstated. By applying ancient wisdom in a modern context, cultivating essential mindsets for sustainable survival, and creating practical survival kits based on time-tested techniques, we can empower ourselves and our communities to thrive. The legacy of our ancestors serves as a powerful reminder of our innate resilience and interconnectedness, guiding us toward a more sustainable, fulfilling future. As we embrace these ancient teachings, we not only honor our past but also pave the way for a more resilient and harmonious relationship with the world around us.

Made in the USA
Las Vegas, NV
07 November 2024

11252305R00096